C000299370

Test tubes and testosterone

Copyright © Michael Saunders 2011

All rights reserved. No part of this book may be reproduced or transmitted in any form or by any means without written permission of the Publisher.

Published by Nell James Publishers
PO Box 588, Chorley, Lancashire PR6 6FZ, UK
www.nelljames.co.uk
info@nelljames.co.uk

British Library Cataloguing-in-Publication Data
A catalogue record for this book is available from the British Library.

ISBN 978-0-9567024-1-8

First published 2011

The Publisher has no responsibility for the persistence or accuracy of URLs for external or any third-party internet websites referred to in this book, and does not guarantee that any content on such websites is, or will remain, accurate or appropriate.

Note: The advice and information included in this book is published in good faith. However, the Publisher and author assume no responsibility or liability for any loss, injury or expense incurred as a result of relying on the information stated. Please check with the relevant persons and authorities regarding any legal and medical issues.

Printed in Great Britain.

Test tubes and testosterone

A man's journey into infertility and IVF

Michael Saunders

NELL JAMES PUBLISHERS

For Hayley.

Contents

Author's note

Allow me to introduce myself. I am a man in his mid-thirties. My wife has no fallopian tubes, my sperm are rubbish and yet our two year old daughter is currently trying to use the computer I am typing on to look at pictures of herself on a bouncy castle.

How did this happen? Well …

Introduction: manliness and infertility

In order to understand the process of IVF and my journey through it, I think it is important to visit the psyche of the average bloke and their attitudes to all things regarding fertility. In order to illustrate the point, I would like to take you back a few years to a pub in London.

I had popped out after work for a quick drink with some of the people I worked with. The only thing that marked this evening out from any other was that it was only women and I that were out. I am not saying I was there as some kind of token bloke or gay substitute: it was just one of those things. All was fine as we chatted about work, bitched about clients and generally talked the way we usually did. The lack of men meant that the conversation was reasonably free of football and breasts and as we moved onto the third drink of the evening the conversation turned to babies: who had them already, who wanted them and who was unlikely to ever get any as their partners were always too drunk or never there. Now a man with more foresight than I may have been able to see where the conversation was heading and make some hastily manufactured excuse to leave as soon as possible. I, for my part, was not paying complete attention to what was occurring and so was caught unaware when one of the women from the accounts office announced that she was going to be starting IVF in a few weeks.

I was in my early twenties at the time and the conversation that followed, featuring as it did quite graphic descriptions of drug taking and a far too in-depth analysis on her husband's sperm count, made me feel uneasy to say the least.

I have to say that I was surprised by my reaction. Why should it be that the subject of underperforming sperm should elicit such a response? I liked to think that I was a man of the world. I had done all the things that manly men should do and many of the things that not so manly men should do too. I would have thought that somewhere in the experiences of my past, something would have occurred to equip me to deal with the subject that I bravely ran away from that evening in the pub. The thing is, the conversation I ran away from would never happen if it were a group of men sitting there nursing drinks and contemplating their day. Although sperm may feature indirectly in many conversations that they would have, the actual quality of a particular man's sperm would not come into question and any chap who fancied broaching the subject in polite company would either be laughed at or greeted with a deathly silence as those around him watched the tumbleweed roll across the bar. This is not because men are not interested in such things (we can be as sympathetic as is required, with a modicum of mickey taking), but more than this, the quality of a man's sperm is something we do not like to think about.

A few nights later, I was sitting at home flicking through the hundreds of available television channels only to find that there was nothing on worth watching, when I started thinking. What if I had the same problem? What if I was not firing on all cylinders? To be honest, the idea scared me. I had no particular desire at the time to father children but for some reason the idea that my little swimmers may not be doing what they should terrified me. If you will bear with me briefly while I indulge in a little backyard psychology, I shall endeavour to explain why this may be.

Many years ago when I was in infant school there were two main insults among the kids. The first was to make your right hand flop while slapping it with your left, all the while sticking your tongue behind your bottom lip and saying 'Nerrr! My name's ... (insert the name of the person you are picking on here)' very loudly. The second was to be referred to as a 'Jaffa'. Now the 'my name is...' insults I understood from the start. They were not nice and certainly not politically correct, but they were clear enough to me regarding the insult being made. The Jaffa remark though had me confused. It was some time later when I plucked up the courage to admit to another lad that I had no idea what it meant (but I was pretty sure it was nothing to do with the orange and chocolate cakes of which I was so fond of). The boy I asked, a chap called Gary, simply said one word.

'Seedless.'

When this occurred, I was about seven years old and had no idea at all what this meant. The only thing I knew was that being seedless was obviously a very bad thing and I certainly did not want to be such a thing. Could this prepubescent crudeness be behind my reaction to the fertility conversation in the pub? Well, maybe, but surely every guy I know can't have been in the same boat at school.

Whatever the cause, it still remains that as a species men do not feel comfortable admitting that they have anything less than a fully functioning reproductive system. Whereas women are often more than happy to talk about their inner workings, men will do everything in their power to keep off the subject. We are more than happy to joke about it in a generic way but not happy in the least to get down to the nitty gritty of our own bits.

Another thing to remember here is that male fertility appears to be decreasing with each generation. I am statistically less fertile than my dad and he was less fertile than his. Now these statistics may well be complete rubbish, as many statistics often are, but they are worth mentioning. There have been no recent comprehensive studies to date to back this up but the beginning of this research seems to be a paper published by some Danish scientists back in 1992, which had the sensitive title of 'Evidence for decreasing quality of semen over the past 50 years'. This paper was based on other people's studies, which happened to contain sperm test results for around 15,000 Danish men. From this information, the paper drew the conclusion that the average ejaculation size had dropped, as had the number of actual sperm contained within it. Other studies have taken this information and run with it, often pointing out that each generation is, on average, having fewer children than the one preceding it. Some of these studies lay the blame firmly at the feet of the men. They say that we have less sperm than our fathers did and that is why we are having fewer children. Now you may think that there are many other factors that affect the number of children a couple will have. Social constraints, health and economical conditions could all easily play a part in this but they are rarely mentioned.

One of the first things that occurred to me when I was reading about this was that as it only takes one sperm to fertilise an egg, does it really matter if there are only 30 million sperm making the attempt rather than the 35 million that my grandfather could manage? Unfortunately it does matter. Now you may look at the lady in your life and figure that the sperm really does not have that far to go. I mean she is probably less than 6 foot in height and they do not have to travel anywhere that far. Unfortunately, it is all down to scale. Sperm really are very small. I mean, you may think that a grain of salt or the attention span of a reality show contestant is pretty tiny, but it would be huge to a sperm.

To put it into a human scale; imagine that you live in London and have to get to Glasgow by foot in a week. Simple you may say. It would be hard and my feet would ache but it is certainly something that could be done. Now try it if you have no feet, and no legs for that matter. Now imagine that you are getting weaker by the day and there are lots of things trying to kill you along the way. If you do manage to get there, you are exhausted and dying. You then discover that someone has built a huge wall around the city that you have to break through using nothing but your head.

Not as easy as you first thought, eh? So basically the more sperm you start off with, the better the outcome.

The thing that really struck me though is that I had absolutely no idea how many sperm I had and whether those that I did have were any good. Assuming that there is at least a grain of truth in the studies and their conclusions, I can deal with the fact that my sperm are not as good as my dad's sperm were. If I choose to put my faith in the statistics that say I will have less children than my father then there may be a problem. I am an only child. So less than that would be none. At the time of these thoughts I had no immediate plans to have children and, in fact, no one to have children with. I therefore did what most men do in these circumstances: I forgot all about it and went to the pub.

1. Why choose IVF?

The way that the world generally works is that you go through life meeting various women. Sometimes you end up together; sometimes you do not. Always at the back of your mind is the thought that if she gets pregnant you are in trouble. Then you meet someone who you can imagine having a baby with. Great. Brilliant. Off you go then.

For an increasing number of couples these days, at some point down the line they will have what is known as 'The Conversation'. Both of you will sit down, often to a nice meal and all will be going very well indeed. The man of the relationship will have a feeling that he is onto a good thing here and possibly wish that he had put his best pants on that morning instead of the slightly unpleasant but nicely comfortable ones that he is wearing. The woman on the other hand, will know that there is a reason why they are sitting down to a lovely meal and it is nothing to do with the imminent removal of the man's under garments. At some point during the meal, the woman will steer the conversation towards having babies. The man will think that all is still going to plan at this point and may even consider suggesting something a little risqué. He had better hope that he keeps his suggestions to himself because the next thing that his partner says will be along the lines of,

'Well, it's not working, is it? I am not pregnant.'

The next stage of 'The Conversation' will depend on the mindset of the woman in question and, to a degree, on the man's reaction to her opening gambit. It could all be very pleasant and touchy-feely, or it could be full of shouting and blame slinging. One way or the other, the pants that the man is wearing will become far less important than he felt they were when he first sat down to eat.

Many people have what the medical profession helpfully describe as 'unexplained infertility'. In fact, most infertility is unexplained until such a time that the appropriate tests are done to allow it to be explained. It can be down to a chemical imbalance, an allergy, something physically not working or one of many other things. It is also human nature to seek out someone or something to blame, so if things are not progressing as you would like, it is vital to get yourself and your partner tested for the obvious things that could be going wrong. From a male point of view, it could be something as simple as a particular food that you are fond of yet is adversely affecting your sperm's ability to go in the right direction. If you have some*thing* to blame then hopefully you will not be tempted to blame some*one*.

I was lucky in that my wife and I never had that conversation. We knew that we could not have children the traditional way and also knew that many current fertility treatments would not do a thing for us. Before we met, Hayley had fallen pregnant only to find that the resultant embryo had not managed to make its way from her fallopian tube and into the uterus before embedding itself and settling down to grow. This ectopic pregnancy obviously had to be removed before it ruptured her tube. Luckily it was at an early stage and was removed without any major damage to the tube. In fact she was told that no lasting damage was done and the tube should continue functioning normally. She did not feel that it was the end of the world or even the end of her chances to be a mother. She still had one tube that was working properly and one that should be fine. It may mean that it would take a little longer for her to fall pregnant once she started trying in earnest, but a little time was better than no chance at all. It was something we discussed when we got together but as I said before, I was not consciously searching for a mother to my future children so it was not something I found overly worrying.

After we had been together for a little while, she fell pregnant again. Having had one ectopic, she was looking out for the signs of another. Following a period that lasted two weeks and was accompanied by mounting pain, she took a pregnancy test and shared her fears. I have to say that I had no experience in these matters at all so all I could do was take her to the hospital. The hospital staff prodded her around and took some blood before announcing that she was pregnant and as she had had one ectopic previously she should come in for a scan in one week's time. We took their advice and went home. After a night of no sleep and a little internet research on both our parts, we decided that a more forthright approach was needed and so headed off to the accident and emergency department and told them that we needed to be scanned there and then and that we were not going to take 'no' for an answer. After much grumbling and moaning, the hospital eventually agreed to scan her and we were taken upstairs.

After only a few seconds, the sonographer found the pregnancy lodged in the fallopian tube. The tube was already starting to rupture, so my wife was rushed into the operating theatre as any delay would put her life in danger.

As I sat in the waiting room with my mother-in-law, I tried to work out how I felt about the fact that I was nearly going to be a dad and more importantly, how I felt about the fact that I was not actually going to be one after all. By this time I had only had two days to get used to the idea of parenthood before it became apparent that things were not going according to plan. I say plan, but let's be honest here, it wasn't planned at all. It would have been one of those happy accidents in life.

The operation was a success insofar as Hayley survived and was wheeled back up to the ward where we were waiting for her. As our eyes met she burst into tears and sobbed.

'I can't have babies', she announced.

Whilst hugging her, my mind was trying to work out what this actually meant. The teenager in me was leaping up and down and shouting something about no condoms, but I tried to ignore him and think thoughts that fitted my age and maturity. Up until a few months ago I had been pretty sure that I was not going to have children and I was still getting used to the fact that something had changed inside me. I now found the idea of little ones to be quite attractive. Up until a few days ago I had never even had a close call unlike a few blokes I had known. There was the occasional late period but these eventually turned up and all carried on as before. But the idea that I could actually become a dad had stuck in my mind. Something inside me had been awakened by that positive test result, something that wanted to cuddle, to feed, to chase around and mess about with and generally do all the things involved in dragging a child up today. And now my wife was telling me that babies were out of the question.

Hang on a minute, I thought with a rare moment of clarity, there are two tubes so we should only be down to one even if the doctors could not save the tube with the pregnancy in it. Hayley explained that when she had come around in the recovery room she had asked if they had saved her tube. The nurse simply said 'no'. She then asked if the other tube had been affected.

'Oh no, you have no other tube. If you want children now you are going to have to have IVF'.

I now completely understood the cause of her tears as she was wheeled back on to the ward.

A habit that I have always had, along with many men, is that I want to fix things. Unfortunately, this was not something that could be fixed, no matter how much gaffer tape I had in the loft.

We were now in the same boat as thousands of couples in the UK and probably millions in the world. There are many different routes that people take to end up where we were then. Some have or had conditions that negate them ever conceiving a child, some have poor quality eggs and/or sperm and some have nothing at all that medical science can find and yet are still unable to conceive the traditional way. We had eggs and we had sperm, although no real idea as to the quality of either, and we needed some help in getting the two together.

We figured that the first thing we should do was to look into what IVF actually was. I had heard of test tube babies of course. I was a child of the eighties so it was periodically in the news, often accompanied by someone with unmoving hair who had some argument or other about why babies made in test tubes were evil and should be banned. I can vaguely recall thinking that using that amount of hairspray was far more offensive than a child made in a tube, before my father remembered that there was a programme on giant turtles on the other side and that he had had quite enough of people talking for the sake of talking.

It did not take too long for us to discover that test tube babies are not, and to the best of my knowledge have never been, made in a test tube.

In Vitro Fertilisation (IVF) is something that sounds simple when written down but has taken many years of work and not a small amount of luck to get where it is today. The 'Vitro' part of the name comes from the Latin meaning 'glass', which may be where the whole test tube thing came from. In reality, the sperm and the egg get together in a petri dish, but there is a fair amount of terribly clever things that need to happen before that moment arrives.

For those that are interested, a chap called Patrick Steptoe, a gynaecologist born in England back in 1913, had a theory that the actual act of human fertilisation could be achieved outside the body. All he needed was an egg, some sperm, a pot to put them in and some liquid to allow the sperm to move. This did present a few issues of course. While sperm were easy to come by, or at least easy to procure a donation of, live human eggs were a little trickier to obtain. Most women expel one every month but by the time they come out they are not really very useful and I don't imagine anyone wanted to root around in the toilet bowl to find them. So, assuming that the theory was sound, Steptoe set about working out how to procure a mature egg. He pioneered a technique called laparoscopy, where a long, thin telescope using fibre optics for light was inserted into the body through an incision made in the navel. Using this, Steptoe was actually able to see the reproductive tract and work on removing an egg. In the mid-1960s, Steptoe teamed up with a chap called Robert

Edwards who was a physiologist from Cambridge University. Edwards had pioneered the fertilisation of non-human eggs outside the body and with the help of Steptoe and his method of egg extraction, they would be able to get a human egg at the exact moment during the monthly cycle when fertilisation would normally occur.

So everything was great then? It all worked without a hitch? Err … not really, no.

Edwards was using human ovaries as a container to attempt to get the eggs to fertilise, but it was not until four years after they met that they managed to get an egg to fertilise and more importantly begin the process of cell division; a process that if allowed to continue would result in an embryo and eventually a baby.

In 1976, Steptoe met a woman by the name of Leslie Brown. She had issues with her fallopian tubes that meant that the eggs could not get from her ovaries to her uterus. In 1977, Steptoe removed a mature egg from her and Edwards fertilised it using her husband's sperm. The egg began dividing and two days after it was fertilised it was placed back in Mrs. Brown's uterus. The embryo implanted and carried on dividing and growing. On the 25th July 1978, in Oldham and District and General Hospital, Louise Brown was born. Once the baby was born everyone decided that they had an opinion on the subject. However, as you are reading this, I shall assume that you have no moral objections to the process and I shall address those that do at a later stage (pp. 132-5).

To summarise, IVF in its simplest terms is where the woman's egg and the man's sperm do their thing outside of the body. The resulting embryo is popped back into the uterus where, if all goes well, it implants and grows into a baby.

Having found all this out, Hayley and I decided something along the lines of 'why not, eh?'

2. The tests

Decision made, come on then… Not so fast. Tests first, excitement later.

Being the kind of person that I am, I wanted to get the process started as soon as I could. Luckily, my wife was of the same opinion and so we trundled off to see our GP. We were living in South-East London at the time and were told that the waiting list for the procedure on the NHS was around three years. This, as far as I was concerned, was not the definition of the word 'soon' that I had been banking on. He had a quick chat to us to make sure we were serious and then put our names down on what I can only assume was a reasonably long list.

Once we got home and sat down with a cup of tea we both felt pretty deflated. I had gone from not wanting children, to thinking I might be having one, and crucially to actually wanting one, to then not having one and now having to wait three years before I could start the process of having one. Basically, this was rubbish.

We did a little internet research on private clinics that offered the IVF procedure and found that if we were to do it in the UK then we would be looking at paying somewhere between four and eight thousand pounds plus the cost of all the associated drugs on top of that. Oddly, I didn't have that kind of money just kicking around. I am a man remember. If I did have that kind of cash there are still many cars and guitars I don't yet own so I imagine I wouldn't have had it for very long. In short, we were a little stuck.

However, we then found a private hospital that was only a few miles from where we lived that offered a 'store card'. It was designed for people without private medical who needed things doing and did not want to go to the NHS to have them done. Crucially, the hospital in question also did fertility treatments and had a pretty good rate of success. Amazingly, the card they offered could be used for such treatments. Baby now, pay later, we thought.

The first thing to do once we had applied and been accepted for the private health store card was to book an appointment with a consultant. We did this in about one minute and then sat back to contemplate what we had done. Well, to be honest we had not really done very much at all. This one little thing we had done had the potential to change our lives forever though, so at the very least the occasion deserved to be marked in some way. A cup of tea should do the trick. That and a stunned silence about what this appointment could lead to.

A few weeks later we arrived at the hospital not really knowing what to expect. I, for one, had visions of sterile white walls, soothing classical music and nurses who spoke with an accent that you could not quite place. It is possible that I have watched far too many James Bond films. Unsurprisingly, the hospital did not resemble a genetic research facility built into the base of an active volcano. Instead it looked like a pop-in parlour, with beige carpets that were dull yet hard wearing, brown chairs that had seen far too many backsides and Radio Kent piped in over the speakers that may have had their day sometime before I was born. It was full of people sporting a variety of ailments and, as far as I could tell, no one else was there for any kind of fertility treatment. Fifteen minutes after our appointment should have started, we were called into a small room overlooking the car park, where a man in his fifties sat behind a desk grinning at us.

'Sorry I am running late,' he announced, 'I have been in Greece.'

Apparently this is an acceptable excuse in medical circles although he failed to specify if he had been on holiday to the country of Greece or if he had spent the weekend dressed in his finest T-Bird outfit, pretending to be Danny Zuko from *Grease* and asking to be told more. Hayley decided it was the former of the two options whereas I would still like to believe it was the latter.

The most incredible thing for me about the whole appointment was that our consultant did not once look me in the eye and say,

'You think you should be allowed children? Dear me no! It's a miracle you can walk and talk at the same time.'

Instead he was very nice, very professional and went through the whole process. Before it had a chance to sink in we were well and truly on the road to IVF.

Personally I left the hospital that day feeling very confused and not a little shell-shocked. Everything seemed straight forward enough and we were told at great length that the process was not guaranteed to work and, in fact, probably would not. This was slightly worrying to me but not as worrying as what I would do if it did work. I know that IVF was our only chance to have children, but what if there was a stigma attached to it? What if it worked and our child was destined for a life of hating itself as well as being hated for the way in which he or she was created? The role of the man in making a baby has traditionally been pretty minimal. Ten minutes of lack lustre effort, a grunt and a sigh, followed by a bout of wind and titanic snoring is generally classed as the way to make a baby. (The men are not usually awake for the part where the lady in their lives lies upside down for half an hour in the belief that gravity will help his sperm go to where she wants them to go.) Assuming it works, the man will make a surprised yet happy face as his partner emerges from the bathroom clutching a home pregnancy test and wearing a broad grin. He will look at the little lines on the test and nod in agreement that she is in fact up the duff. He will try not to mention that she is holding a small plastic stick covered in wee. After a while he will go to classes and indulge in a spot of back rubbing, but he will, for the most part, leave the lady to get on with things.

With IVF, I thought I would get a chance to be more actively involved. Obviously not in actually getting the sperm to the egg, of course, but in other areas such as helping to get Hayley's body prepared, in administering the medication and things of that nature. These thoughts suffered their first set back once we got home from our first appointment and sat down to read the paperwork we had been given. There were pages and pages for Hayley, detailing drugs, timings, hormone levels and much more. I dutifully read through it all wondering where my part would come in. Eventually, towards the bottom of page four was a section for the man. Right, this was it. This was where I started to get involved.

It was quite a small section now I came to read it. It basically said that my job in the whole process was to ejaculate in a pot.

Twice.

And please don't spill any.

I passed this information onto Hayley who thoughtfully produced the pot that would contain ejaculation number one. It was quite a large pot I noticed. Maybe it was designed for my grandfather and his superior sperm. Although probably not, as if the statistics are to be believed there would have been no reason for him to have the pot in the first place.

'When did he say we need to drop the sperm off?' I asked.

'Thursday,' Hayley said, still wiggling the pot suggestively. 'After we get tested.'

I nodded. The testing. Not for fertility, oh no. We had to go and make sure that neither of us had anything unpleasant 'downstairs' and I am not talking about the nasty mirror in the hallway either. We both had to be tested for HIV and Hepatitis.

I have to admit to being slightly annoyed when we phoned the GUM clinic and explained what tests we needed and why we needed them, that they were more than happy to help and told us to pop along whenever we had the chance. I was annoyed because I was imagining that we would have to concoct some kind of story in order to justify the tests we needed. I had stories involving all manner of debauchery gone wrong that I was ready to regale the clinic staff with but, regretfully, none would be needed.

'Now what have you got to remember?' Hayley asked as we arrived at the GUM clinic one chilly morning.

'Hmm?' I asked in a non-committal fashion.

'It's a GUM clinic,' she smiled. 'Not the clap clinic.'

I made a face that I hoped would put across the fact that of course I was not going to refer to it as the clap clinic. I would never do such a thing. Never, ever. Unless it was funny, in which case I may hint at it at some point.

The look on Hayley's face told me that she completely understood what I was thinking and that she was going to hit me with something if I did what she knew I was capable of doing.

We made ourselves known at the desk and sat down to flick through the selection of four-month-old gossip magazines that were piled on the table in the waiting room. I had barely caught up with what Posh and Becks were doing when my name was called and I was ushered into a side office by a female nurse. In the office stood a couch, another door and a middle-aged man behind a desk. He looked up and smiled as he ruffled some papers before placing them back in front of him.

'So, HIV and Hep, yes?' he asked.

I nodded.

'Syphilis?' he enquired, raising an eyebrow.

'Why not?' I replied as the man produced a pen and made a mark on one of the sheets of paper that lay before him.

'Now we need to do a physical examination!' he announced.

'No we don't!' was my reply.

'Oh yes we do!'

'You do realise,' I stressed, 'that these tests are for IVF treatment, don't you?'

The man looked crestfallen and turned to the nurse who had shown me in.

'We won't be needing the examination room thank you nurse,' he said with a distinctly sad tone to his voice.

The nurse turned upon her heel and left the room. It appeared that the doctor had lost interest in me now for he told me to go with the nurse and she would take the required bloods. I thanked him, although my thanks were more for the fact that he had not pushed his evident desire to have a rummage around my nether regions and I dutifully followed the nurse to another room.

The thing about having tests for conditions such as HIV is that you start thinking about whether you may have actually contracted something nasty at some point in your life that you would not necessarily know about. Somehow I had gotten through adult life up to this point without ever having a blood test. I am not really sure how I managed this, as Hayley seems to have had loads for varying reasons over the years. The nurse was lovely and took the blood with the minimum of fuss although she did put an exceptionally large piece of sticky tape over the lump of cotton wool that I was told to press onto my arm to stop the bleeding. It was only once I had left the room that I realised that the tape was stuck to a large amount of my arm hair.

We both decided that we were not going to worry about the outcome of the blood tests and so headed home. I have to admit to spending most of the journey home being somewhat preoccupied about the results that I had previously said I was not going to worry about. I was pretty sure that I had not done anything in the past that could have put me at risk but I have also seen the government advertising campaigns that hint at the idea that most people under thirty may well be harbouring all manner of unpleasant infections. As I had once been under thirty myself, what did I have lurking down there?

In the time honoured British fashion, we got in and put the kettle on. A sit down and a nice cup of tea would do the trick. What it would not solve though was the big issue of how I was to remove the huge lump of tape that was still clinging, limpet like, to my forearm and all my arm hair. I tried gently pulling at it but to no avail. I did note that Hayley had begun to look at the offending piece of tape in much the same way that a cat looks at a distracted mouse. I decided that the best course of action was to take my tea into the bathroom and run a nice hot bath to soak the tape off. Ignoring the laughter from my wife, I did that very thing.

Emerging from the bathroom clutching a now removed and shrivelled lump of sticky tape, I was greeted by the sight of Hayley and the pot we had been given at the fertility clinic. She placed it on the shelf in the bathroom and announced that she had arranged a lift for the morning so the pot needed to be filled before I went to work.

Giving a sperm sample is very simple in theory. The clinic had told us that I had to abstain from ejaculating for between two and four days prior to providing the sample, so we went for the middle ground of three days. That was pretty much the sum total of the instructions that we received. Things of note that were not mentioned: where you should do the deed, how you get the resultant deposit into the pot, whether you are allowed any help with giving the sample and how full the pot should be once you had finished.

My train was at ten to eight in the morning and my mother was due to arrive five minutes before this time to pick up Hayley and the pot and take them to the clinic. So, ten minutes before my mother was due to arrive, my pot and I went into the bathroom to do what we had to do. I tried to think nice thoughts, hoping the cat did not walk in midway, and got down to business.

A few minutes later and the sample was in the pot. I popped the lid on and engaged in a little cleaning up just as I heard the front door open and my mother arrive at the house. We had been told two further things with regards to the delivery of my sample. Firstly, it must be at the hospital within one hour of ejaculation and secondly, it should be kept warm during the journey. They suggested that the pot be wrapped in a sock and popped in Hayley's bra for the duration. I wandered to the bedroom clutching the pot to my chest and found one of my old socks to wrap it in. Hayley, quite rightly, had refused to use one of her socks. I thought that having it wrapped and therefore out of sight would be best because although my mother and Hayley knew what I had done, it was not something I fancied shouting about and certainly not something I wanted on display as I walked down the stairs. Besides which, the pot was hardly overflowing and I really was not in the mood for comments of 'is that it?' and 'would you like to try again?'

Both Hayley and my mother gave me a look known as knowing as I appeared from upstairs brandishing my sock. Hayley took it from me as I rummaged in my bag to make sure I had everything I needed for the journey to work. After a brief discussion, it was decided that there was no way that Hayley was going to travel to the clinic with a pot of sperm in her bra and so it was relegated to her pocket. We both noted that my mother did not offer the services of her bra for sperm transportation and, if I am being totally honest, this is something I will be eternally grateful for. With that, I said my goodbyes and wandered across the road to the train station worrying slightly that I should have at least taken the pot out for a drink and dinner before using it in such a blatant way.

As I sat on the train in the traditional pose of the com-muter (that being the one where I had my iPod on and my face buried in a book), Hayley and my mother leapt into the car and set off for the fertility clinic. As I said before, they had one hour from the sample arriving in the pot to get it to the laboratory. This would normally not have been a huge problem but it was eight in the morning in south-east London rush hour traffic and my mother seems to have an almost pathological desire not to break, or even slightly fracture, the speed limit. Commendable you may think, but also very annoying if you have a pocket full of sperm that is rapidly cooling. There were a few hairy moments and one very shocked old lady who cut them up at a junction and was treated to Hayley winding the window down and shouting about sperm, but finally Hayley, my mum and the little pot arrived at the clinic with a full five minutes to go before the hour was up. A short sprint and a little queue jumping later and the sperm were in the lab and ready to be tested.

For me, a day of reflection and introspection followed. I was still worrying about the HIV test, although I had absolutely no justification for doing so, and now I had my impending sperm analysis results to worry about too. It is not that I am a natural worrier but the results were important to me and they were not something that I could actually do anything about. If either of us had anything nasty lurking in the under carriage then the clinic would refuse to treat us, meaning that children were completely out of the picture. Mind you, if either of us did have anything like that I think children would no longer be our highest priority. The sperm results were not likely to put an end to the whole process but could certainly make things more difficult than I was hoping they would be.

As I said before, it does only take one sperm to fertilise an egg. If you are going for the traditional way of making babies then the more you start with, the greater the chances are that the one you need will actually survive long enough to do what it was made to do. With IVF, however, things are very different.

There are two ways for the egg to become fertilised and both happen within a petri dish. The first way, and the preferred option for me, is that the egg and the sperm are plopped in the dish along with some fluid and left to get on with it. Compared to the journey that sperm have to make inside the female body, this one is very easy. It's just a short wriggle across the dish, head-butt the egg for all your worth and in you go. The second option is called Intracytoplasmic Sperm Injection, or ICSI, and is where a single sperm is picked up in a tiny hypodermic needle and physically injected into the egg. The main advantage of this technique is that it theoretically only requires one good sperm in order to work. So if you have a low sperm count, which is defined as less than twenty million sperm per one millilitre of ejaculation, or if your sperm are not moving in the right direction or at the right speed, then ICSI may well be the way that you can father children. However, there are two negatives to this process as far as I can see. Firstly, and this is very important if you are paying for your treatment, it will cost you around an extra thousand pounds on top of all the other costs that you have. Secondly, there is a chance that the egg will become damaged during the process. Although the needle is incredibly thin, it is still a needle being poked into something that was not designed to have a needle poked into it.

This was one reason that I was being a little paranoid about my sperm results. Another thousand pounds added to our bill would probably not make us abandon treatment but it would certainly mean that if it worked we would still be paying for the child after his or her second birthday. Coupled with that, there are also the niggling thoughts that lurk behind your eyes that you will be less of a man if you have a poor sperm result.

There are a few things in this life that, as a man, you are expected to conform to. You are expected to follow football. You are certainly expected to drink beer and, more importantly, be able to drink it without falling over after two pints. You are expected to be able to fix a car. All of these expectations can be argued against with relative ease. You can site health reasons for the lack of beer drinking that you may indulge in. You may get a few sarcastic comments but nothing with any particular venom. If you can't fix a car, you can draw people's attention away from that fact by being mates with a mechanic or making sure you have a car with a warrantee so it does not become an issue. Not liking football is a bit more of a problem, but with a little lateral thinking, most people will let you off. What happens though if you are a man with poor sperm? What if I am a man who has problems getting his lady pregnant? Does it, in fact, make me less of a man? Well it depends on your definition of what makes a man 'a man'. If you define your manliness simply as the ability to father offspring far and wide, then yes it does make you less of a man. However, if you judge your masculinity on more modern values such as emotional strength, the support you offer to others and your ability to cope under pressure, a poor sperm test result could actually mean that you have to become more of a man.

We had one more test to do before we went back to see the consultant. This one was for Hayley though, so not much for me to do other than try to keep up with what was going on. Before we can start IVF, the clinic need to know roughly how Hayley is going to respond to all the drugs that she will be taking. Basically, the drugs are used to trick her body into releasing multiple eggs at the same time rather than the one per month it wants to release. There is a follicle stimulating hormone (FSH) present in both men and women and the clinic need to know what level this hormone is on day three of the woman's cycle, with day one being the first day of period bleeding. The theory is that on day three, pretty much nothing should be going on in the ovaries and so the FSH should be at its base level. The hormone is produced by the woman's body to trigger the production of follicles and the release of an egg from inside the dominant follicle. As she gets nearer the menopause and the eggs are running out, more and more of this hormone is produced. Any level measured as less than 10 is generally classed as good and should mean that the woman has plenty of eggs. Levels over 10 hints that something may be awry and if you have levels of more than 20 then there could be something more serious occurring.

Seeing as this was just another blood test, I elected to go to work and leave Hayley to it. This was purely out of a sense of duty to the company I work for and nothing whatsoever to do with not wanting to run the risk of anyone sticking more tape to my arm hair.

3. Before you start treatment

It was a Friday. I had the day off work, although I had promised my boss I would have my phone switched on 'just in case'. Today was the day that we visit the consultant once again. It was the day that the results from the Clap Clinic jury were in and it was the day that the Sperm Analysis would be made public.

As before, we made our way to the clinic and took our place on the brown seats in the waiting room. Having learned from my out-of-date gossip magazine experience of last time, I came prepared with a book. Again, as before, we got called in to see the consultant around fifteen minutes after our appointment was due to start.

'Terribly sorry,' he said. 'I have been in Greece.'

Hayley and I looked at each other and smiled. I was still not sure which Greece (or *Grease?*) he was referring to but in my mind his statement only added weight to the idea that, in his time off, our consultant was in fact Danny Zuko, aka John Travolta. Minus the looks, acting ability and personal airliner of course.

First item of business, after we had all exchanged pleasantries, was the blood test results. First in was HIV.

And our survey says …

No.

Excellent news. Neither of us had HIV. I am still not sure why I found this such a relief, but I guess I must have been entertaining the possibility that the result was going to be bad news. Still, nothing to worry about from that one.

Next were the results from the Hepatitis jury.

Mr. Saunders. Nil points.

Mrs. Saunders. Nil points.

Hurrah. It would appear that whatever we have both got up to in the past is not going to come back and haunt either of us in a scary way. This could well call for a cup of tea. Except we are in a private hospital and I doubt very much if anything comes for free around here. I am slightly surprised that someone does not come in once you have gone, measure the indentation in the chair you have been sitting on and send you a bill for the difference in dent between when you arrived and when you left. Anyway, there was no time for either tea or billing speculation, for the next item on the agenda was my sperm.

Obviously I put a brave face on it, but I have to admit that I was slightly worried. I knew I had sperm and I had a rough idea that at least some of them were functioning correctly as I had been responsible for Hayley's second ectopic pregnancy. But that was not proof by any means that they were the thundering warriors of reproduction that I was hoping they would be. I wanted them to be charging across the petri dish, little sperm-sized swords in hand, like something from *SpermHeart – The Movie*.

Who was I kidding?

'Well Mr. Saunders,' began the consultant. 'Good news. You have around forty eight million sperm in your sample.'

Now that really was good news. Whichever way you look at it, that is a lot of sperm.

'Motility was good.' The consultant continued.

So basically, they were all moving around like… well, like sperm I suppose. Bless my little wriggling swimmers, all forty eight million of them.

I must have been grinning because our consultant chose that moment to bring me back down to earth.

'However,' he said, adopting a tone that could only be described as boding, 'only twenty per cent of them are travelling in the correct direction.'

Houston, we have a problem. So if we do a little maths here and work out that I have nearly fifty million sperm, but only ten million of them know where they are going, that means I have a comparatively useless amount of good sperm. The consultant said there was probably enough for me to conceive naturally but that it would be very hit and miss.

To sum up, I have a lot of sperm, all of which are charging about like lunatics. The issue is that although they all get ten out of ten for enthusiasm, only a few of them get any marks at all for direction. Based on these numbers, it seems rather surprising that they managed to find their way out of my testicles and into the pot in the first place.

One thing was still bothering me. How do the people that test the sperm know which direction they should be heading in? I mean the sperm are all in a dish. Not the most natural environment for them you may argue. I assume they don't have a large picture of an egg on the wall and then count the sperm that head in that direction.

I stopped thinking silly thoughts for a moment as our consultant was trying to explain something to us. He was saying that because my sperm were rubbish and could not be relied upon to find their way from one side of a dish to the other, he would recommend that we went for an ICSI treatment. He explained that one of the best-looking sperm is selected and physically injected into the egg. He explained further that this would be done by a bloke called Steve. He ensured us that this was a fully trained embryologist and not just some chap called Steve that he happened to meet in the staff canteen.

As I sat and pondered the condition and general lack of enthusiasm of my sperm, the meeting progressed on to the next point. That being Hayley's FSH level.

'Seven point eight,' the consultant smiled. 'Very good.'

As I said, anything under ten means she still has plenty of eggs left, so seven point eight hints that her ovaries are still nicely stuffed with eggs.

The meeting finished with us being given a list of drugs and being told that we would get a call when the hospital had worked out a start date for our treatment. Given how the meeting started, the end was a total anticlimax. We thanked the consultant, wished him well for his next trip to Greece and left the hospital in silence.

'So that's it then?' I asked. 'We just wait?'

Hayley nodded. 'Rubbish, isn't it?' she said.

We arrived home and flopped straight down on the sofa, both of us feeling pretty deflated. After all the build up we were now simply expected to wait. The main question was, how long would that wait be?

It was a question that was to be answered the following day and the answer was about four months. Four months? I guess it is only natural that there would be a bit of a wait, as the clinic needs to schedule in every part of the process, including the bits that only matter if the treatment is a success. Apparently our consultant was going to be in Greece for a whole month during our wait, which although it did not come as much of a surprise, did slightly annoy me. However, as there was nothing at all that we could do about it, we decided to just get on with life and wait.

This worked for one entire day, as the next day the paperwork arrived to remind us exactly what we were doing and to poke fun at us because we would not actually start doing it for months. Not that we actually have to do much with the paperwork, as most of was to be filled in with the nurse when we get our next appointment through.

With the paperwork put somewhere safe, well somewhere that Hayley could find it at any rate, we tried to put things to the back of our minds once again. Again this only lasted for one day as the clinic called to arrange an appointment for us with the nurse. This was where we went through the paperwork and had every stage of the process explained. It was in a little under a month.

Now we had a definite date when we had our next appointment, although no date yet for actually starting treatment. We decided, yet again, to carry on as normal.

One day later, the list of required drugs arrived from the hospital. I will go more into the whys and wherefores later but there are a lot of drugs involved in the whole IVF process and they can cost an awful lot of money so bear with me for a moment. There are several options with the drugs. If you are having treatment on the NHS then the drugs will be given to you free of charge and all you need to worry about is what to do with them, something we shall come on to. If you are paying for your own treatment then the bill for the drugs is likely to come as something of a shock. Some clinics will sell you the drugs but it is definitely worth contacting the company that makes the drugs and asking if they sell direct. Many do and you should find that the price goes down by a substantial amount. It is still likely to be over a thousand pounds but it could be twice that if you buy through your clinic. Some clinics do not mark the drugs up and some will even order them on your behalf directly from the supplier.

We actually found another option. Because we had signed ourselves up to the NHS waiting list in our area, and more importantly been accepted, our GP found a little loophole in the legislation. He found that you were entitled to one treatment and one lot of drugs for free. There was nothing to say that you had to use the drugs for the free treatment. Now, this loophole has now been closed, at least in the area we were in, but it is still a question worth asking before you start. So, having found this out, we trotted along with the list of drugs and the address of the clinic and consultant and were given our prescription, which we took to the supermarket pharmacy straight away.

As the story stops for a few weeks at this stage, it may be a good time to mention something that affects a lot of people at this point. By the time many couples get to the stage of being accepted for IVF, they have been trying for children for quite a while and wanting children for much longer. This is often more applicable to women, but the effects can be felt and often have to be dealt with by the men. Imagine years of sadness, frustration and disappointment that have been put aside and pushed to that space in your head where all the nasty thoughts reside. The hope caused by a late period, followed by the sadness as the period finally arrives. The excitement after every time that you may have made a baby and the feeling of that excitement collapsing as you realise that, yet again, it has not happened this time. Now imagine that you are offered a way to put that behind you, to finally conceive the child you have wanted for so long. Now imagine that you have to wait for several months. The dangling carrot is on a very long pole indeed. Imagine all these things and you can see that it is often the case that people are not at their most emotionally balanced as they wait for treatment to begin. It may well be the case that as you go about your daily lives, the lady in your life starts to act in what you could describe as a slightly odd fashion. They could well become incredibly moody, withdrawn, bad tempered and generally grumpy. There is also a very real possibility that they will burst into tears upon every sighting of a baby or in some cases a pushchair. As far as I can tell there is nothing you can do should this occur and the best you can hope for is that it will pass with time.

Time. It's a wonderful thing time. It can heal all wounds apparently. It can take you on wonderful journeys and it can drag forever if you are in a school assembly. Time is a good thing and it's even better when you use it to surf the internet and record things from the telly.

To that end, I can remember getting home from work one day to discover that Hayley was looking very pleased with herself. A quick trip to the kitchen to make a cup of tea led me to discover several pots of vitamins on the worktop where once stood a bottle of wine from the previous night. Someone had also stolen the tea and replaced it with the caffeine free version. I wandered back into the lounge where Hayley was sitting to be greeted by the legendary line.

'I've been looking on the internet...'

Good grief. I did not need to be a genius to work out that Hayley had discovered that things like zinc, calcium and vitamins C and D could help fertility. I could also wager a guess that she had found out that alcohol and caffeine were bad too. I had not been to the fridge yet but I knew it now featured lots of healthy food, including things high in iron and full of goodness. I must have let out a sigh because Hayley asked me what was wrong. The truth is there was nothing wrong at all. I loved the fact that she was doing all of this. There were limits though.

'Where's the proper tea?' I asked.

She laughed. 'In the cupboard behind the plates.'

To be fair, and leaving the tea aside for a moment, Hayley did have a point. There were things we could both do to increase our chances of success. From a man's point of view, all we really have to worry about is making sure that the sperm that we have are in the best possible condition. They need to be leaping around in a very enthusiastic manner and, perhaps more importantly, leaping around in the correct direction. It's all very well if they are all charging around but if only a few have the right map then it is not going to do any good at all. First and foremost on the list of things that Hayley found for me to follow were the things I was not allowed:

Alcohol.

Cigarettes.

'Recreational' drugs.

Caffeine.

Fatty foods.

Tight trousers (and anything that could crush or over heat your man parts).

To take them one at a time then. Staying off the booze is a fair enough comment really. We all know how drinking too much makes you feel the day after. It fills your body with toxins, dehydrates you and generally makes your immune system fall apart. It is only logical that if you feel a complete state then your sperm are not going to be in tip-top condition.

Now for the fags. Fun though they may be, they also fill your body with toxins, mess around with your chemical balance and generally make you slowly fall apart.

Now to the recreational drugs. As I am sure you have heard at some point in your life, drugs are bad. You may argue that they do have up sides but be that as it may you are putting unnecessary chemicals into your blood stream, which are going to do your sperm no good whatsoever. Essentially, all alcohol, all cigarettes and all recreational drugs have nasty chemicals in so if you want to get the best out of your testicles, avoid all as much as you can.

Now fatty foods may well also contain some nasty chemicals, but the main issue with them is the fat. I am sure that you have seen graphics on the news of clogging arteries and although it takes time to get to that stage, too much fat does affect the blood-flow around the body and therefore to the testicles, and if they don't get enough blood they will only produce feeble sperm.

Caffeine is not something that needs to be completely avoided, at least not in my life, but it is something that acts as a stimulant and so should be kept to a minimum.

Avoiding tight trousers is a far more sensible suggestion than it may seem. Ignoring the fashions of the day and the advice of people with silly names on the telly, tight trousers as well as tight underwear cause the temperature of testicles to rise and unfortunately they do not work well when hot. There is a very good reason why they dangle about, which is to allow the temperature to be regulated. It could also be to give members of the opposite sex a good laugh but I feel that is more of a by-product rather than the main reason. You have to remember that your testicles are amazing things. They produce massive amounts of sperm over their lifetime, pretty much on demand (rather than those ovary things that only manage to release one or two eggs a month). Each individual sperm contains all the genetic information from you that your future children will ever need. They are great things, so look after them. I am not saying you should polish them every Sunday or anything, but remember that they are almost too important just to stuff in your pants and forget about. Besides which, the only reason for tight trousers as far as I can tell is to try and make yourself attractive to women, and if you are going through IVF then the chances are that you already have one women who wants to breed with you and that should be enough for anyone thank you very much.

To summarise: don't eat rubbish, don't drink rubbish, don't put nasty things into your body and make sure you have happy knackers.

Most people who go down the IVF route find that they have a fair wait between being accepted and starting treatment. Many women find that they have to go on the pill in order to regulate their periods and some just find that they have to wait for a slot to become available at the clinic. Either way, the chances are that you will have some time on your hands. Now I know that IVF is stressful and expensive but try to remember that there is a chance that it will work and if it does there are certain things that you take for granted in life that will not be possible, at least for a while. One of these is foreign holidays. It is not that pregnant women are banned from aircraft or that small children explode at 30,000 feet, it is just that you will have so much going on and an IVF pregnancy is somewhat different to a traditional conception. If time and funds allow I think the best thing you can do is go away for a quiet week or two in the sun. By quiet I mean a holiday where you sit around the pool sipping chilled fruit juice rather than one where you sleep all day because you got so drunk the night before. Although there is no medical evidence to back it up, I firmly believe the best way to start IVF is to be as relaxed and chilled as possible.

We decided to go away on a cheap package deal, although we did make sure that it was one where no young children were allowed. Hayley had been bursting into tears more and more while we waited for treatment and often had to be dragged past baby shops to stop her from going in and crying over the tiny socks. We packed our bags, with maybe a couple of extra factual books than we would usually pack, and headed off.

We returned from our drink-free holiday feeling slightly more relaxed than we did before we went. We only had a week to spend kicking around the house before we could go back to the clinic for our next appointment. Hayley was not handling the waiting very well. As far as she could see, she had made the decision to start, we had been accepted and she did not want to wait. We had a little issue with her period though as up until now her cycle had been anywhere between thirty and thirty five days long. This month though it decided to be exactly twenty-eight days long and finally do what it was supposed to do. This was a good thing, as the clinic definitely prefers you to have standard length menstrual cycles. It was bad news for Hayley though as for some reason it came with the worst period pains that she had had in a very long time. This only served to put her in a worse mood and heighten the sense of guilt that she was feeling with regards to how quickly we got on the road to IVF. Although she was grumpy about waiting, she also felt incredibly bad about being grumpy because so many people had to wait months if not years to begin their journey. I did what all men should do in situations such as this. I dropped her off at her mother's house for the evening and watched a rubbish film with space ships in it, until it was time to get back in the car and go and get her. It seemed to work, as she was far better once we got back to the house.

Finally the day arrived for our appointment with the nurse. It had only been a week since we had come back from the sun, but that week seemed to drag forever. Luckily, Hayley was getting her hormones under control and we had even managed a trip to the shops without any tears, although I definitely saw her eyes welling up when a lady with twins passed us on the way to the car park. We got up as normal and trundled around making breakfast and drinking tea, but I don't think that either of us was particularly hungry. It was just something you did to distract yourself from what was going on. It was not that something bad was occurring, far from it. It was just the events of today could dictate our entire lives from this point forwards.

After a while we both had to admit that we really could not drink any more tea and it was time to be going. Our appointment was the first of the day at the clinic so the drive there was through south-east London morning rush hour traffic. The journey was unusually silent as we crawled along the roads.

After much grumbling about the traffic, we finally arrived at the clinic and sat down upon the brown chairs. The nurse arrived a few minutes later and called our names. This time we did not go into the little room by reception that we had been in before, and thankfully the nurse did not claim anyone had been to Greece recently. We were lead down several corridors, up a short flight of stairs and finally up one floor in the smallest lift I have ever been in, before being asked to go through the third door on the left. This we did and sat down on the two seats on our side of the desk. The nurse took her seat, produced a file of paperwork and smiled. The smile was a good thing, for now it all got a bit serious. We made sure that all was correct on our papers regarding our names, address and so on. There were a few questions that I think were designed to find out if we were mentally unbalanced, but were not exactly challenging to answer correctly and then we got down to business.

The first thing was to go through the drugs, which are done in a number of stages and although the actual drugs used will vary from woman to woman and from clinic to clinic, the principles are the same. Firstly, the woman will need to take something to stop her menstrual cycle in its tracks, which is known as Down-Regulating. In Hayley's case these were to be administered nasally twice a day. One sniff in each nostril, twice a day. This sounded quite simple and Hayley seemed happy with the idea. The nurse then showed us a dummy bottle of the drug we would be using to down-regulate so we could take a look and have a play with it. We were on a drug called Synarel, which tricks the pituitary gland into not releasing the hormone that is required to trigger ovulation. You have to start squirting this up your nose on the first day of your period and keep going for as long as you are told too. In our case, Hayley had to keep squirting for twenty days. On the twentieth day, we would have to go back to the clinic for what is known as a Baseline scan. This is to check that your body has down-regulated correctly. If it has not, then it is not the end of the world, it may just require a different dose of the drug or a change in prescription.

Assuming that all is going to plan, you then move onto the next set of drugs. These are not as simple as bunging something up your nose. Oh no, these chappies have to be injected. There are two different ways of administering these. The first is the traditional method of a little glass bottle containing the drug and a syringe. You suck up the correct dosage into the needle and away you go. The second option, and luckily the one that we were given, was a devise that looked like a fat pen. You click a tiny needle into the bottom of the pen, twist the top until it says the correct dosage, stab yourself in the tummy and press down on the end of the pen. Again there are numerous drugs that can be used. The one we got was called Gonal-F, which sounded terribly medical to me. We were told to take this for twelve days during which time Hayley would have three scans to check on her progress. The idea is that this drug tricks her body into producing multiple eggs, which can then be removed and introduced to my sperm in a controlled environment. These eggs will be contained in little fluid filled follicles. Unfortunately, the clinic can only tell how many follicles there are: they have no way of knowing how many of them contain eggs until it gets to the time when the follicles can be drained. They then have to have a rummage around in the drained fluid and see what is in there. Before the eggs can be removed though, you have to have one last injection of something called Ovitrelle, from a needle that looked far bigger than the Gonal-F one, in order to mature the eggs for removal exactly thirty-six hours later.

The final drug that Hayley had to take was something called Cyclogest and came in the form of a pessary. For those that do not know, these are little bullet shaped things that are designed to be pushed where the sun does not shine. The nurse said that ideally they should be taken vaginally but if Hayley found that to be a problem then she could take them anally. This seemed to me to be a fancy way of saying that if she didn't like it she could shove them up her arse. So much for the bedside manner.

Having had the drugs explained, the opportunity to play with the injectors and mused upon the size objects that would have to be inserted in the opening of Hayley's choice, we moved onto the way that things work inside the female body. It is important to note at this point that I went to an all boys' school and our sex education mainly consisted of one word:

Don't.

With a note to the effect that if you 'do' then bad things would happen so please make sure you got the young lady's name. I think there may have been a government scheme at the time that banned schools from mentioning anything that could be classed as remotely 'icky'. Following the nurse's chat, and a few hastily drawn diagrams, I felt I suddenly had a much better understanding of how things worked. It is not something I am going to go into now but I would recommend that it is something you research before you start treatment as the way things actually work and the way they are explained in school textbooks are not entirely the same.

Next on the agenda were my sperm results. I got the feeling that this could just be adding insult to injury, but I sat there like a good little boy and took what was coming. The long and the short of it was that I now had someone else telling me that my sperm, although plentiful, were rubbish. It turns out that only nineteen percent of them had even a vague idea where they were going, rather than the twenty percent I had previously been lead to believe had a map. The nurse was a little vague herself about how motility is actually measured, but it would seem that as long as a sperm is moving forwards then it is classed as going in the right direction. What this would appear to mean is that the majority of mine were spinning around in circles, charging off to whence they came or doing the reproductive equivalent of leaning on the water cooler chatting to the girl from accounts.

However, this was not the end of the matter. When a man ejaculates, there is far more that comes out than just sperm. In fact some people produce no sperm at all while still managing to ejaculate. The seminal fluid, as it is known, usually contains sperm but it also includes various enzymes and fructose that provide nutrients for the sperm on their journey as well as a medium through which they can swim. However, when your sperm are being used for IVF, their needs are very different to those trying to survive inside a woman. As there is nothing trying to attack or kill them and they have considerably less distance to cover in their petri dish, they do not need this food supply. There is also artificial fluid in the dish to allow them to swim to the egg so they don't need their own liquid in order to move about. This means that the sperm can be removed from the fluid. In some cases, mine included, the sperm are just not quite able to move through the seminal fluid to any great degree. This could be because they are a little weak or it could be that the fluid is just too thick for some reason. For the sake of my own self-confidence, I have chosen to believe that, in my case, it was the latter. When you provide your donation for the clinic, the sperm are cleaned. They are stuck in something resembling a tiny but incredibly powerful washing machine and spun until the sperm and the fluid separate. Once they are separated, the measurements are taken again. Without all that gloopy stuff, my motility improved from nineteen percent to ninety per cent. Now here is where we enter tricky ground. My un-washed sperm results were pretty rubbish which means that I met the criteria for ICSI, where a single sperm is injected into the egg to fertilise it, but my washed and spun sperm results were good and left to their own devises would find and fertilise the egg themselves. The clinic we were at based their decision of whether to do ICSI or not on those initial unwashed results. At the time we did not know any better and so we agreed, despite the fact that it was going to add over one thousand pounds extra to our overall cost.

One thing that I found exciting, although I am still not sure why, was that we got our own needle bin. It was yellow and could only be disposed of by incineration. It made me feel like a very high-class drug addict. It is simply not the done thing to throw ones empty skag needles in any old bin, you know?

The biggest news from this meeting though was that they finally gave us a start date. Well an approximate one at any rate. They said that Hayley should start the nasal spray on the first day of the period after her next one.

We got home and sat down with the traditional cup of tea. The conversation in the car had been very superficial as if both of us were trying to avoid what was a very big subject. The weirdest thing for me was that I could finally visualize Hayley being pregnant with our baby, my baby. My own flesh, blood, neurosis and chins. This was a really big thing for me. Up until now I think I had been trying to avoid this line of thinking in case the treatment did not work and all I was doing was setting myself up for a very big fall. Before today's meeting it was as though the whole thing was happening to someone else, but now it was starting to hit home. We had played with the drugs and been told when to start using them. Basically, in a few months time, Hayley could be pregnant. This is both exciting and scary as hell if I am being honest. I am completely unprepared for all of this so I think it may be time for some more research. The odd thing is I couldn't help feeling the whole IVF thing is far more of an adventure than other people have when they go down the traditional route of baby making, which seems to involve there being nothing on the telly at Christmas and a newly emptied drinks cabinet, resulting in a birth sometime in September. I am not knocking this method as it worked fine for my parents, although my dad never could bear to have any Advocaat in the house after I was born. Part of me feels that the excitement of being able to say 'was that the one?' after you have made love is not as much fun as really being involved with, and fully under-standing, the process of fertilisation. I am hoping that the journey of IVF is something that both Hayley and I can really share: well, both of us and my pot of course. Part of me feels I should ask for the pot back so that I can show our future child how it all started. Part of me knows that the whole thing is unlikely to work though. I mean, what are the chances of someone being able to remove an egg, bung a sperm in with a needle and shove it back in so Hayley's body does not notice and turns it into a baby? Only one way to find out I guess and that process would start in a little under two months.

It was not a restful night for me after we had our meeting with the nurse. I can't say that I was particularly worried, but my brain took it upon itself to keep producing random memories at thoroughly inappropriate times. For some reason it seemed to think that a detailed memory of riding across the lounge at my grandparents' house when I was four years old was a worthwhile thing to mention. Admittedly, I was on a bright orange tractor but I failed to see the significance of this. My brain then moved on to more obscure things and by the time it was three in the morning, I am pretty sure it was just making things up to annoy me. Mind you, maybe once upon a time I was a unicycling penguin and I had just forgotten it. After this point I abandoned all hope of a good night sleep and opted for wandering the house to try and find something to do that was boring enough to send me to sleep. Late night telly should do the trick, I reasoned, pouring myself a soft drink and settling down with the remote. It only took a few minutes for my brain to realise that the late night poker show was not going to occupy it for long so it started thinking again. This time though it was slightly more useful. It started coming up with images of Hayley in a maternity ward. It was hazy on the details but there was certainly a little baby involved.

All this late night or early morning silliness did serve to highlight a couple of important points though. Firstly, it seemed that I could finally imagine the birth of my own child and secondly, I had no clue what birth actually involved. If the television were to be believed it mainly featured a lot of screaming and blame slinging, but I knew enough to know that things seen on the telly should be treated with cynicism at best and outright hostility at worst. I left for work that morning with a plan.

By lunchtime I was distracted from the plan by tiredness and my body doing some very odd things. Now it may well have been the lack of sleep, but my stomach felt bloated, my back and ankles hurt like hell and if I did not know better I could have sworn I was craving a *Pot Noodle*. We had not even taken a single drug on the road to possibly pregnancy and yet my body had decided to give me sympathy pains. The swollen stomach could have been the late night soda I guess and maybe lack of sleep was contributing to the aches and pains. There really was no excuse for the cravings though. Luckily, I had a half-day so I headed home with a view of putting the plan into action.

I may be giving the plan too much of a sense of grandeur here. It was more of an idea really. I felt that I needed to see a real birth. Not a sanitised, pre-watershed 'scrubbed to within an inch of its life' birth. You see, I had been trying to think about birth during the day and as far as I could tell, I had the idea that it is all very clean and smell-free. There may be a certain amount of screaming and yelling but it is all done with a laugh and a smile. There is a faint popping sound as the midwife dons a baseball mitt and hurls herself across the room to catch a wonderfully clean and sparkly baby, who gives a little cry and then smiles as he or she is handed to their glowing mother. Having explained this theory to Hayley, she replied in a way that should not come as too much of a surprise.

'You pillock!' she said. 'Get the computer on.'

I did as I was told and soon we were looking at several rubbish and out of focus birthing videos on a well known video posting website. The thing is though I grew up in the 1980s. I am a child of the MTV generation. Poor quality and out of focus just does not cut it for me. I need the full bandwidth, high definition, surround sound, Dolby encoded, one hundred frames a second cinematic experience. It was a shame that 3D television was so rare at the time as that would have certainly done the trick. I have a sneaking feeling that I am quite well prepared for the whole IVF side of things but that I was not at all prepared for the birth. Well, this was about to change.

As they are so fond of saying in American sit-coms: Oh my God! Or, if you are of the texting persuasion: OMG! Or if you really want the truth: OMFG!!!

We went out and bought a birthing DVD. A proper camera-up-the-bits kind of DVD. There were several very scary things about this. The first one you notice is that it was filmed some time ago, certainly before any kind of pubic trimming became fashionable to do. Even before you saw anything regarding actual birth, the whole area in question looked like a hedgehog in a road accident. The doctor in the video had one of the most impressive moustaches I have ever seen, and amazingly, the woman in labour still seemed to be taking him seriously. Once I had stopped laughing at these things, we finally got around to the point of the film. After much pushing, huffing and not a small amount of cursing, the baby's head could be seen nudging its way out into the world. Hayley explained that this was called crowning just before the dull voice-over told me the same thing. All of this was all very fine and good. (The thing that prompted the outburst at the top of this paragraph was just coming up.) The woman appeared to be pushing and huffing and doing everything that the moustachi-oed doctor said she should. Unfortunately, the head was not coming out as it was supposed to. So the doctor took a pair of scissors and snipped the skin below where the baby's head was stuck. Not an 'excuse me madam' or a 'do you mind if I do this?' Not a bit of it! Just grab some scissors and away you go! Hayley reacted as you would expect as the very loud, surround sound pop reverberated through the lounge. She crossed her legs, yelped and turned away from the screen. For my part, I simply sat and stared, struck dumb by the sight and sounds in front of me. Surely there was a more pleasant way of dealing with this problem? I know that it must be inevitable that, once in a while, people have to give birth to a baby with a head that is bigger than the exit, but just attacking with scissors cannot, surely, be the only option? I voiced these opinions to Hayley who said that it often is the only option and apparently the women who have had it done are usually so distracted by other pains or so dosed up on drugs that they do not notice. Once all was said and done, the woman on the video gave birth to a small, wrinkly thing that she seemed very pleased with indeed.

I have to admit that the whole thing was pretty amazing, if a little unpleasant, but it was not as disgusting as I had feared. I was still not sure about how I would feel about seeing my wife in that position, and more importantly, from that angle. Part of me feels that the Victorians had the right idea whereby the husbands were not allowed in the delivery room at all. They were confined to the waiting room where it was their job to pace the floor awaiting news of their offspring's arrival into the world, at which point they would produce cigars for themselves and anyone else who happened to be in the room with them. Of course, in those enlightened times, the health benefits of smoking were widely acknowledged and encouraged. In these times though, it is simply not done for a man to pace around in a little side room. Oh no! He is expected to take a full role in the proceedings. In many cases simply being in the room is not good enough either. He has to get down the action end and witness the birth of his child. He has to see the wonderful moment as the head pops out of his wife's lady parts. The very same lady parts that he is trying to think of as attractive and not a rather shocking looking thing that a baby is passing through. He often has to cut the cord, which does not cut as easily as those television programmes would have you believe. Having done all of this, he is then passed a child that is often screaming and almost always covered in stuff that he does not want to think about. He then has to make coo-ing noises and be all 'new man' about the whole thing when he would much rather be passing around cigars, safe in the knowledge that he will not have to have any contact with his child until the baby has been well and truly cleaned with all unpleasant smells removed.

Having come to the end of the birthing film, or at least the end for now, I wandered in to the kitchen to do the manly thing and put the kettle on. Upon my return I found Hayley rummaging through the Sky guide and pressing the record and series link buttons with much gusto. It seemed that my televisual experience of babies and birth had only just begun.

It was the next day when the fruits of Hayley's button pressing were made apparent. I returned from work and flopped down on the sofa with a view to killing at least an hour watching something to do with cars when the remote was removed from my hands and I was presented with a list of things that had been recorded in the small hours of the previous night. It would seem that several of the channels with the high numbers that I do not usually go near had been having something of a baby themed night. Programmes like *Test Tube Babies*, *Baby Story*, *Portland Babies* and *Extreme Pregnancy* had all but filled up our planner.

'What do you fancy watching?' Hayley asked.

'*Top Gear*?' I ventured without much hope of a successful outcome.

'We have *Test Tube Babies*', Hayley continued as though I had not spoken, 'or how about *Dangerous Births*?'

I guessed that the titles of these shows pretty much told you all you needed to know about the contents of the programmes. The test tube one sounded like it might be worth a look. After all, we were about to have a go at making our own test tube baby, even though it was actually a petri dish baby, so it might be worth seeing what other people had gone through to get theirs.

The people they featured on the show had generally been through a lot, far more than Hayley and I had at that time. They had couples who had been trying for children for years and years without any success at all. Often these people were having IVF as their last go at getting a baby. Although I tried to be my usual cynical and aloof self, many of the stories were heartbreaking and after the first episode it started to make me realise that there were many people in a far worse situation than us. It did not slip my mind though, that we did not really know what our situation was with regards to IVF. We knew that we had been accepted, but as we were paying for it ourselves that was not altogether surprising. What we did not know was how successful any treatments may be. It could be that we would be one of those couples that have many goes at IVF over the years, racking up more and more debt to pay for it and never getting the child they are increasingly desperate for. I figured that line of thinking was not going to do me any good at all, so I got comfortable and sat back to learn what went on during IVF.

Two hours later, I made the executive decision that it was definitely time for food and wandered off to get a takeaway with stories of infertility still buzzing around my head. As I have said before, the whole wanting children thing was still relatively new to me and the idea of not being able to have them was even more recent. I could not begin to imagine what it must be like for people who have spent their whole lives wanting nothing else but to have children of their own. For many of them, IVF represents the last bastion of hope and possibility, which I guess is the same for us except that we haven't been trying for our entire lives.

Enough of this, I thought. Time for chips.

As time marched ever onwards towards the arrival of Hayley's period before the start period, things got more strained in our house. Hayley was definitely grumpier the closer the date she was due to come on came. She started to brood more and more on the reasons behind our infertility. In some ways it was good that we knew exactly why we could not conceive traditionally, but in other ways it was not so good as it allowed there to be blame.

Personally, I felt that the two ectopic pregnancies that Hayley had were something that could be chalked up as 'one of those things', but as we got closer to the start Hayley started to get angry at the hospital for the way they treated her and the way she found out she could not have kids. The anger then turned to worry about what would happen if the IVF worked but the pregnancy got lodged in what remained of her fallopian tubes. If this were the case then the doctors would almost certainly have to remove what remained of her tubes but there was also the very real possibility that they would have to remove considerably more, meaning that there would be no future possibility of children unless we went for surrogacy or adoption. Hayley even said she knew she was being silly and the chances were that this would not happen but she could not help worrying. I did what I do at this point every month in Hayley's cycle, which was to keep as far out of her way as I could. There were tears and tantrums, there were grumbles and stomping. It was only the open plan nature of our house that prevented the door slamming. Soon, and not a day too soon, the period arrived. This is known to Hayley and her friends as Aunt Flo, or AF for short. This was new to me as I thought that Aunt Flo was a character from *Bod*, the 1980s children's show.

We were now officially in our last 30 days before treatment. There was only one thing to do and that was to try and clear the planner of all the baby programmes that were residing there. We had been avoiding them while Hayley was going through the tears and tantrum phase, but now the programmes were back on the cards again. My routine for the next 30 days was this: wake, work, home, watch baby programme, bed.

Within two weeks of Hayley's period before the final period starting, I had seen programmes that covered how babies are conceived, how they are conceived with a little help, how they are conceived with an awful lot of help and how they come out. We also covered what happens if they don't come out and what happens if they come out too fast or too slowly. We watched things on people having babies in hospital and at home and one with a reconstruction of what it may be like to give birth in a bus shelter. Essentially, I was happy that I understood the theory behind babies and everything that goes before them and immediately after them: the thing that was starting to worry me was that I had no actual practical experience of them. If the treatment was successful, and at the moment I liked to believe that we had as much chance as anyone else of it working, then at some point in the future we would have a baby and quite frankly I had no bloody clue what to do with one.

4. The treatment

As the date of Hayley's possibly final period arrived, things were getting tense again. There was a small amount of tension regarding the fact that we could actually be on the baby road any day now, but far more was coming from the interesting hormones that course around the female body in the few days before their period starts. Hayley was not at her most balanced and the trepidation of finally starting treatment was not helping. I did not say as much but I also felt that the amount of baby programmes that she was watching were not doing anything to alleviate her mood. As I said before we had overdosed on things like *Test Tube Babies* and *Bringing Home the Baby*, but the programme we watched most was *Portland Babies*. This was an old reality show (I am guessing it was old based purely on the quality of the programme and the hairstyles contained therein) that was set in the Portland hospital's delivery suite. It mainly featured rich foreign women with ugly husbands screaming their way through labour and, in Hayley's opinion, generally making far too much fuss about the whole thing.

We had dropped the prescription for the IVF drugs into the supermarket chemist a while ago and a few days before the period arrival date was due, we got a call telling us that the drugs were in and we could pick them up whenever we wanted. We did that very thing straight away. There was a brief discussion regarding the Cyclogest pessary prescription as the pharmacist claimed that they were only for women suffering from PMT. We simply gave him one of those looks and he stopped venturing opinions and put them in the bag. As we got back in the car, we both had the most stupid grins on our faces. It really felt like we were one step closer to starting.

On the day that Hayley's period was meant to arrive, we were in the supermarket. We did not need to buy anything but it was a way of distracting ourselves from what we were about to do. As it turns out it was a very bad way of distracting ourselves as the place was full of people with babies. I say people, but that may be too kind a term. They were people insofar as they had arms and legs and so on and so forth but they mostly had the one same thing in common. They were all wearing tracksuits and not one of them looked like they had done anything involving exercise for at least ten years. All the babies appeared to be called Chelsea and most were being screamed at by their mothers. Needless to say, we both made a very sharp exit from the shop wondering if the amount of leisure wear that you own is directly proportionate to your ability to breed. I ventured that it may have something to do with the large gold hoop earrings, but Hayley claimed they are purely circumstantial. The reason I mention the visit to the shops though is that something monumental, at least to me, happened in the car park. We had unwittingly parked near the parent and child spaces and as we were returning to the car we saw a woman unloading a small baby from its car seat and trying to strap it in to its buggy. Trying being the operative word here, as it looked more like she was trying to get a fair sized squid into the harness. The monumental thing though was that the child was very cute. I said as much to Hayley and she burst into tears. She later explained that it was partly because there were so many babies around, partly because she was so hormonal but mostly because it was the first time I had ever admitted to finding a baby anything other than 'icky'.

By the evening there was still no sign of the period although we were now at the point where Hayley was crying at pretty much anything. So as not to dwell on it, she put another baby programme on as I started to drift off. No matter how many of these programmes I see and how much I understand about the inner workings of the female reproductive system, I still can't help but think that the whole conception thing is very badly designed. I was beginning to feel sorry for the sperm of people who can conceive in the traditional way as the poor little things stand almost no chance at all of getting where they are going. Obviously, my little swimmers stand even less of a chance what with there only being about half a dozen of them that know where they are going and even they would probably get tired before they get to where they are meant to be, coming to a staggering halt in the lower part of the uterus and doing the sperm equivalent of milling about a bit. IVF really was a very clever thing if it could provide the help that my little chaps needed to actually fertilise an egg.

As the baby programmes came to an end, we made our way up to bed. Hayley had a major sulk on when she emerged from the bathroom so I did not have to ask if her period had turned up. She grumped around the bedroom for a while, occasionally swearing at inanimate objects before finally getting into bed. She was still mumbling as I fell asleep.

The next day was much of the same, as was the next. On the third day after her period was meant to have arrived, Hayley declared that we were going to a funfair. I think she was trying to scare her period into starting. It did not work and we returned home without anything bleeding but with two extra furry toys that we did not really need.

'Bloody pants didn't work,' was Hayley's cryptic offering as we walked back to the house. I made puzzled sounding noises and she explained that she had her best white knickers on so that her period would start as it always does when she has white pants on. There was not really much I could say to that.

It was dark. It was the kind of dark that tells your body, on a subconscious level, that the thing to be doing is sleeping. Sleeping and dreaming, and not having to think about waking up for hours and hours. What the dark is definitely not telling you to do is to wake up to the sound of a toilet flushing and someone putting the bedroom light on. As I tried to persuade my eyes to peel themselves open, I heard a very excited shrieking sound. In order to justify my reaction, I would like to point out again that it was the small hours of the morning. I had been asleep and it was very dark outside. I was not thinking about my life outside of the rather nice sleep I was being raised from, so I turned over, pulled a pillow over my face and pretended to be asleep.

Hayley removed the pillow with a flourish of her wrist and grinned at me.

'It's here.' She said in a manner not dissimilar to the little girl form the poltergeist films.

What's here? I thought. Certainly not sleep that's for sure.

I sat up. 'What?' I managed, rubbing my eyes and vaguely wondering where my pants were.

'Period!' Hayley almost screamed.

'Ah,' I said having found the missing underwear. 'Tea?'

She nodded and headed off towards the lounge. There are very few things that a man will consider to be an acceptable reason for waking him up at this time of the morning and most of them are negated by the arrival of a period. Having said that, once I had remembered what my name was and what I was doing here, everything slotted into place and I realised that this was a pretty momentous moment. One that I would not enjoy, or possibly remember, without considerably more caffeine inside me.

With the tea made, we both sat down on the sofa. I clutched a mug of tea and Hayley clutched a little cardboard box. With a grin, she pulled the box open and took out a slip of paper from within. She read for a few moments and then announced that the nasal spray that she was about to remove from the box could cause headaches, vomiting and hair loss. After pulling a very unhappy face, she read on to the section that said that these side effects were 'very rare' and calmed down again. Surely it would make more sense that the little message telling you that side effects are very rare to appear *before* the list of possible and vary rare side effects so the reader does not panic about bits of themselves falling off as soon as they take something? Anyway...

Hayley got the little spray bottle from the box and we shared a look. The look said, get the camera you fool, this needs to be documented. I took the hint and decamped to the kitchen to rummage through the man-drawer to find the camera. Duly found, I returned to the sofa and my tea and prepared to shoot.

Hayley pulled a variety of faces as she posed with the spray before finally squirting it once up each nostril. I got several action shots, safe in the knowledge that when you are having IVF it is the one time that it becomes socially acceptable to show your children pictures of their conception. And that was that all done. Back to bed.

In many ways IVF is harder for women and this isn't just because they are the ones taking the drugs and have people poking around in them. As I have said before, there is an awful lot of waiting around and this gives more than enough opportunities for analysis, soul-searching and introspection. In the couple of months leading up to the first great squirt, we had both spent a reasonable amount of time both together and separately, thinking about things. Hayley had obviously decided that she had had enough of such things and that she needed something to distract her from further fretting. So when I arrived home from work a couple of days after we had started squirting, I found Hayley in the spare room surrounded by steam and wrestling with some-thing that resembled an octopus while poking at the wall with a small plastic knife. I articulated my thoughts quite succinctly.

'Err... What?' I asked eloquently.

As the steam cleared to reveal that the octopus was in fact a wallpaper steamer, Hayley smiled coyly. 'I thought that yellow might be nice.'

I made vaguely positive mumbling noises, raised my eye-brow slightly and took myself off in the direction of the kitchen, figuring that Hayley would potter down sooner or later. The sound of the boiling kettle did the trick and a very smelly and sodden Hayley emerged from the spare room. I handed over the tea and said that I thought yellow was a lovely idea and would she mind if I sat down for a while as I had been at work all day. She said that would be fine and trundled off once more to continue savaging the wallpaper.

Left alone with my tea and thoughts, my mind finally began to relax and I started to think about things. I felt it was obvious how Hayley was feeling about everything, or at least obvious that she wanted something to concentrate on to stop her thinking about everything. The question I wanted an answer to was how was I feeling about it all. I sat and thought for a while as I flicked idly through the television channels and came to the conclusion that the whole thing had so far failed to sink in at all. It did not feel real yet, but I think that may have been because I did not have anything much to do at this point. It had only been a couple of days and a few sprays, which Hayley had done herself. I felt rather excess to proceedings. This was not something I was going to dwell on because I figured that Hayley had quite enough to contend with without me getting all grumpy because I wanted to do more. Besides, if I said something I am sure that she would have found me lots of jobs that needed doing.

Before I continue, I should probably go into a little more detail about the drugs that Hayley was currently taking. Synarel contains an active ingredient that is pretty much unpronounceable to anyone without a medical degree, although if you fancy a go then it is called Nafarelin. What this very clever little thing does is to affect the pituitary gland in the brain. Now the pituitary is basically the bit of the brain that controls the production of some hormones and stores others until they are needed. The amount of the drug that Hayley was taking would eventually cause the pituitary to stop producing the follicle stimulating hormone (FSH) and the luteinising hormone (LH) completely. The latter hormone is the one that triggers ovulation and the former is the one that triggers the production of the follicle that will eventually contain the egg. However, as the production of these two hormones reduces to zero, the production of oestrogen also drops meaning that the lady taking the drug goes through a shortened version of the menopause. Anyone who has been around someone who is going through the real menopause will know some of the effects that this produces. The charitable person would say that is causes women to become slightly irrational and a little tearful. If you were not feeling quite so forgiving, you may possibly venture the opinion that the women become complete loonies who will burst into hysterics at the drop of a hat.

I had done a little research on Synarel beforehand and so was expecting, if not totally prepared for, what happened on the fifth day after we started. The lovely sweet girl I was used to coming home to had seemingly been replaced by a wailing banshee. In the space of about ten minutes after getting home from work I had made the tea wrongly, not cleaned up a mess that I didn't make, breathed too loudly and I think I was told that I got up in an incorrect manner that morning too. The bedroom appeared to have changed colour since I left it that morning although admittedly it was an improvement so I was not complaining at all.

There was light at the end of the grumpy tunnel, although I was still not convinced it wasn't an oncoming train. After I had admitted blame for all the things I had or had not done, Hayley calmed down and announced that she had booked a series of acupuncture sessions. We had asked at the clinic as to whether this was likely to help the treatment and they had said that it might, or might not, but as there is no documented scientific evidence one way or the other they could not say for sure. My personal feeling is that anything that helps you relax is generally going to be a good thing. There are a lot of stresses that go with fertility treatment and a little chill time is never going to hurt. Unless, of course, you are the kind of person who relaxes by getting drunk and beating up cloakroom attendants. I decided that the best course of action for the immediate future was to keep a low profile and try not to do too many wrong things.

The next day was Saturday and the first of Hayley's acupuncture sessions. We both popped along to what looked like a disused shop and rang the bell. As we were waiting for what seemed far too long a time, Hayley went a very funny colour and started sweating. After she had removed as many clothes as was socially acceptable, she cooled down and the door to the acu-puncture 'clinic' was opened by an oriental chap in a cardigan that he must have obtained from my late grandfather. We were ushered inside whereupon we were greeted by an old lady who appeared to be chewing something that was not meant to be chewed. As she did not speak a word of English, cardigan man asked us some questions and reported the answers back to chewing woman. After a fashion we managed to get across that we were having fertility treatment and did they think this was something they felt they could help with. Chewing woman stopped chewing for a moment and made a gesture that could possibly have been interpreted as a nod. Fair to say Hayley was not brimming with confidence as she was lead into the backroom while I was shown to a chair that must have been at least as old as the woman and told to sit and wait. Part of me was tempted to wander off and have a look around the shops while Hayley had her session but I was not entirely sure that I would be allowed back in again and I had a sneaky feeling that if I left they would either try and sell Hayley or force her to take ownership of a small furry gremlin, that she would definitely feed after midnight and then it would all go spectacularly bad. So I stayed and read the badly translated notices as many times as I could to try and kill the time. There was not even a gossip magazine from the turn of the century in the waiting area, which was odd as up until then I thought there was some kind of European Union directive to make sure that this was never the case.

I heard Hayley explaining, once again, what it was that she wanted from behind the screen door. I heard no reply but was told afterwards that the old woman simply smiled and started poking needles into places where Hayley was reasonably sure they should not be going. However, whatever the old woman did it seemed to have a slightly relaxing effect on Hayley. This was tested as soon as she left the treatment room as cardigan man started going on about the healing and helpful nature of certain herbs. After a while we agreed to take some herbs home and look at them even if we did not crush and boil them as we had been instructed to do. Cardigan man finally opened the front door and we emerged, blinking, back on to the high street.

After a little window shopping and a spot of tea and cake we headed home. There was decorating to do but the first thing on the 'to do' list was to have a look at the herbs we had been carrying about. We opened the bag and found … Well, it looked like a bag of daffodil bulbs and not very healthy looking bulbs at that. They looked like they had been kept in an airing cupboard for three years before someone had the great idea to put them in a bag, claim they had healing powers and flog them to unsuspecting saps who would buy anything as long as the man in the cardigan would just agree to open the damn door and let them out again.

We crushed the bulbs and chucked them into a saucepan filled with water, turned on the hob and left them to it for a while. If you want to know what our kitchen smelled like fifteen minutes later when we went back in then I can only suggest that you move into a packet of dry roasted peanuts that has previously been inhabited by an elderly Yak suffering from terminal flatulence. Full marks for bravery go to Hayley though as she strained the tea and poured it into the oldest and most unloved mug that we had. She held her nose and downed half the concoction. And that was that. The rest of it went down the sink and we both left the kitchen, having made sure we opened a window first.

'I really hope this is all worth it.' Hayley said as she flopped onto the sofa.

Six days later, twelve more squirts and one failed attempt at drinking the daffodil tea, although this attempt did involve loading it with cinnamon and nutmeg, and we were off to the clinic for our scan. This is known as the Baseline scan and is done so the clinic can check that the Synarel has stopped everything that it should and also allow them to see what Hayley's insides look like when they are not too busy doing stuff. The scan was an internal one which, for those of you who are not familiar with it, involves sticking something that is roughly the same size and shape as an old policeman's truncheon up Hayley's lady parts. This scans straight up into the uterus so the doctor can have a good look and make sure that nothing is occurring that should not be. From our point of view, we got a lovely look at Hayley's insides. Once the doctor was happy, she removed the probe and sat us down for a chat. Luckily, it was a good chat and she said that we could start the next round of drugs that evening.

All systems go then. Tally ho and all that. Actually, that is not quite right. The Gonal-F drug is taken by injection and as neither of us have ever been diabetic or a drug addict, we had absolutely no experience whatsoever of injecting either ourselves or someone else. Our experience went as far as poking an empty injector pen into an orange during our 'practice the drugs' meeting, which was actually quite a while ago now I come to think about it. We got out our instructions and laid everything out on the coffee table. Hayley took up the injector pen and held it aloft. For reasons that are still unclear, we both burst out laughing and so she put the pen down again. We took a minute to compose ourselves and Hayley took the pen up once again: less giggling this time which we both found encouraging. After a little fiddling, she took hold of a pinch of flesh from her tummy and aimed the needle.

Deep breath …

The needle bounced off her skin and caused more childish giggling from both of us. We soon regrouped and Hayley pinched once again. This time she managed to draw blood before putting the pen down and looking sheepish.

'We need ice,' she said.

Taking my cue, I heaved myself from the sofa and plodded to the freezer. Here I discovered a small issue in that we had no ice. I was left with the choice of either trying to scrape some ice from the side of the freezer and hope I got it back to the lounge before it melted, or I could borrow a trick that my father used when he was in the St. John's Ambulance. I duly got a sandwich bag from the cupboard and a handful of frozen peas from the freezer. Peas in bag, bag duly tied and we were ready to rock. Or ready to numb may be closer to the truth. I appeared, triumphant, in the living room and waved the bag of peas at Hayley. She was not entirely complimentary about my makeshift compress. In fact she said,

'What the hell is that?'

'Peas. Trust me it'll work.'

'Hmm,' was all the reply I got but being determined, I pushed on.

Hayley took the peas and held them on the side of her tummy while I had a little fiddle with the injector pen, as she had decided that it was now my job to do the stabbing. Hayley looked away and …

Twist, pull, squirt. Twist, pull more, stab, hold, squirt, pull and breathe. Nice.

As I pulled the needle out Hayley asked if I was in yet. We shared a look but both of us resisted the urge to fill the resultant conversational gap with any crudities. Once the needle was out and deposited in out high class drug addicts needle bin, we noticed that the hole I had left was bleeding more than either of us had expected. Hayley even got a trophy blood stain on her grey tracksuit bottoms, although she would like it stated that she does not wear them out and only had them on at this point as she had got mud on her jeans. We carefully put the drugs back in the fridge and the needle bin back in the cupboard and then sat back down to think about what we had done. This lasted about three seconds until Hayley remembered that we had a chocolate cheesecake in the fridge and that she had not had a cup of tea in nearly two hours. Again I took my cue and supplied both.

The next day Hayley went back for another acupuncture session, which she reckoned did make her feel more relaxed. Although they did not try and sell her more dry and dusty bulbs, they did make her feel bad for not drinking her bulb tea as often as they thought she should. As such, she returned home and started crushing and boiling. I popped briefly into the kitchen, took one breath and decided that there was something important that I should be doing in the garden. I returned an hour or so later to find that Hayley was painting another wall and her bulb tea was still sitting on the kitchen worktop in a distinctly un-drunk fashion. In fact all it appeared to be achieving was prolonging the smell.

After dinner and some relaxing, the time for the injection had arrived again. We both went to the kitchen to get the stuff that we needed. As Hayley opened the fridge door, all the lights went out. We both stood still, partly to see if they would come on again and partly because we could not see a thing. After a few seconds, Hayley closed the fridge door and we both swore. It seemed that standing in a pitch black kitchen was not going to make the lights come on. We had a couple of problems here. Firstly, we had to get the next injection done and secondly, the drugs had to be kept cold so if the power stayed off for too long the fridge would cease to be cold and the drugs would be ruined. It was clear we needed a plan. It was clearer still we needed a torch.

I heroically produced my mobile phone from my pocket and flicked it on. Okay, it was not the Wembley Stadium flood-lights, but it did allow me to see a couple of feet in front. I found Hayley and made sure she was safe, before heading outside to the granny annex where my parents lived. I could definitely see light coming from one of their windows so it looked as though the power cut was only us. Typically there was no moon, so I picked my way along the path using the mobile for light. I returned to the house a few minutes later to report that my parents had light and a working fridge. As the torch was somewhere in the garage and neither of us fancied going to find it, we bagged up Hayley's drugs and took them over to my mother's fridge. My parents vacated the kitchen to allow us to do the drugs in peace and, after I returned to the house to get the peas, we did that very thing.

Another five days, five injections and two more failed attempts at drinking the foul tea later, we had arrived at our first follicle scan day. After seven days of the Gonal-f, Hayley's body should have started producing little fluid-filled follicles that would, hopefully, contain eggs. In order for the clinic to ensure that this was happening at the correct rate and that the dosage of the drug was accurate, we had to go and be scanned. Well, Hayley had to be scanned. I simply had to drive the car and try to make sense of what I could see on the screen during the scan. We headed off early just in case of a traffic mishap, with Hayley declaring that she had to have 'relaxing' music on in the car, to which she promptly fell asleep, and we slowly made our way to the clinic. As we did not have to see our consultant for the scan, we were called in precisely on time.

It was another internal scan which can't have been nice for Hayley but she was relaxed about it and the doctor soon found our first follicle. After a few minutes, she found that Hayley had four good-sized follicles in her right ovary and three in her left. There were lots of little ones too but the doctor said that these could either grow or shrink so it was not worth getting too excited about them just yet. She noted that there were around fifteen smaller ones and said she would check again when we came back for our second scan. The other thing that the doctor had to check was the lining of Hayley's womb and whether it was starting to thicken. This is important as it is within this lining that the fertilized egg will nestle and grow assuming that everything works. If the lining is not thick then the embryo will have nothing to stick to and will, more than likely, just slide out again.

The drive home was not pleasant for Hayley; she had been feeling tender for the past few days and was definitely starting to look bloated. The internal scan must have irritated something that was already tender. We stopped a few times and even popped into the services for tea, finally making it home in one piece. On the plus side though, Hayley's emotional state seemed to be calming down as it was now two whole days since we had any tears.

We continued as we had been for the next three days. There were injections and baby programmes and many cups of tea. Hayley was getting increasingly tired and irritable, although I think the grumpiness was more to do with being exhausted and bloated than any hormonal imbalance. On the third day, we were back in the car and off to the clinic again. As Hayley was so tired, we went for the relaxing music once again but she completely failed to get any sleep as she was finding it increasingly hard to sit comfortably. At the clinic it was someone we had not met before who was going to do the scan today. The lady looked pleasant enough until you attempted any kind of conversation when it became obvious that she had no sense of humor whatsoever. Hayley was not impressed at the idea of this humorless woman sticking things in her bits but as we needed the scan and there was only one doctor at the clinic, we had little choice. Once we got into it though, the doctor was professional enough and she quickly found the area she should be looking at and announced that Hayley had eleven follicles in each ovary, so twenty-two in total. Of these twenty-two, the doctor said that at least eleven of them should be of a suitable size to contain an egg when we came to that point in the treatment. Although no one at the clinic ever really said how many follicles we should be expecting, they all seemed happy with what we had. There was talk before we started of something called Ovarian Hyper-Stimulation Syndrome, which is where the drugs have too great an effect and the woman's body starts producing too many follicles and possibly eggs. Although many women undergoing IVF will show signs of minor OHSS, these symptoms will generally ease, although some will find that they produce dangerous amounts of follicles and eggs and there is a chance the treatment will have to be stopped. Happily, Hayley's follicles are all within the recommended limits, so that is all well and good and back in the car we go.

I have noticed as we go on through the treatment that I seem to have an inability to think more than a day ahead of where we are. I know that the reason I am stabbing my wife every night with a needle is so that her body will produce multiple eggs. I know that the reason we need those eggs is to try and get one or more of them to fertilize with my rubbish sperm. I know that, assuming this occurs, we will have one or two fertilized eggs inserted back into Hayley and I know that she needs to carry on with drugs to help these embryos stick to her uterus. I know all these things. I also know that there are terrible things going on in the world all the time. All these things I know and none of these things I seem able to think about. I can think as far as the following evening when I know I have to do the injection. When we are driving to the clinic, I am able to think about how many follicles I hope Hayley will have. I hope that when the time comes I shall be able to concentrate on what is occurring during egg collection. I hope I can do what I need to do when my pot and I are lead to wherever it is that we have to go. I hope all of these things but I don't know them. I am not sure if it is as a direct result of this, but my behavior seemed to be getting increasingly bizarre. I have started putting my face to Hayley's stomach and singing things like 'grow little eggies'. What is worse is that Hayley has started joining in. I even found myself giving her ovaries a stern talking to the other night to try and persuade them to produce a nice amount of follicles and not too many. We only had three days until our final scan so it was probably about time that I got my brain to accept what was going on and look at the bigger picture.

That night, Hayley admitted that she was finally getting excited about the whole thing, although it might have been that she was excited to be nearing the end of the injections. In less than a week from now, if all went well, she would have real baby embryos back inside her. We would not know if they were going to turn into actual babies, but they would be in there at least. In three weeks time, she could be proper pregnant. As was fast becoming a family tradition, we sat down and had a look through the baby programmes that we had recorded the previous night. Quite why they are on at silly times of the night I have no idea, but there you go. I have to say though, that I actually started enjoying them more than before as all the little science bits now actually applied to us. Even the stock footage of an egg being injected with a sperm that they show every damn episode now means something more. I am still getting slightly annoyed by the incredibly low production values and the fact that the voice over appears to have been done by a chipmunk. Luckily, the people on tonight's show had a successful outcome, as I really do not think that I could watch people failing in IVF right now. It is not that I am in denial, of course, but something is telling me that I have to keep positive. That same something is also telling me that I cannot talk about it. I have to believe that every stage of the treatment will be a success, but I also have to keep quiet about those beliefs. I have no idea why I feel like this but I do, so I am just going to have stay quiet and keep positive.

Three days, three stabbings and no more foul tea later, we were back in the clinic for what would hopefully be our final follicle scan. We had little miss grumpy knickers again but she must have been on some kind of medication as within a few minutes of us getting to her room, she smiled. I was waiting for her face to crack but no such entertainment was forthcoming. She was even apologetic about what she was about to do to Hayley's bits and actually used the warm gel. Anyway, Hayley still had eleven follicles on each side and all looked big enough that they could possibly contain an egg. They were ranging in size from about 12mm all the way up to 23mm. The formally grumpy doctor said she was happy and we now got to move onto the next stage. She said all this once she had removed the probe from Hayley of course. She also explained again what the plan would be. We would be booked in to have Hayley's eggs extracted in two days time. The operation would be at half past eight in the morning. The doctor said that the final injection had to be administered exactly thirty-six hours before extraction, not thirty-seven and not thirty-five, but thirty-six, exactly a day and a half before. I think that the doctor was really trying to hammer home the importance of the timing of the final injection but she did go on a bit. We said we understood and that we could be trusted to get the timing right and that we would even set an alarm to make sure that everything went according to plan.

Every time we left the clinic I found myself in a slight state of numbness. So far, it had always been good news and although I was being very quietly optimistic, it was still a shock when it actually worked. In my heart I knew we would get a good number of follicles at the right time and we would move onto the final injection, but there was always the chance things would not go right. There was the chance the follicles would collapse or there would be so many of them the cycle had to be stopped. Both of these are quite rare, but it still came as a surprise when neither of them happened. So this was very nearly it then, with only one more injection to go. Should we do something to mark the occasion? Tea and cake it is then.

One more stabbing and then that is it. As half past eight approached, we got the final injection needle out and made our way to the sofa. This one was not the nice, easy-to-use pen that we had been using for the Gonal-F injections, oh no! This one was a proper syringe, with a little bottle of liquid that you had to suck up into it. As was now the tradition, I got comfortable and then had to get up again to get the bag of frozen peas. I passed them to Hayley and attached the needle to the syringe. I will admit to a slightly shaky hand as I drew the Ovitrelle into the syringe. I squeezed the air out exactly as the nurse had showed us, then held it up to the light and gave it a gentle flick. We had not been told to do this but I have seen *Casualty* and if it is good enough for them …

Hayley held the peas on her tummy for a while as I took up position to her right so as to get the best stabbing motion.

'Ready?' I asked.

Hayley nodded and removed the peas. She looked away, as had become her wish, and I firmly pushed the needle into her skin.

Or not, as the case in fact was.

The needle bounced. I saw her tummy indent as I pushed, but I did not even break the surface. I regrouped, had a sip of tea and made my apologies. Hayley put the peas back and we had another go. With exactly the same results.

I stood up and started to walk around the room still holding the syringe. It looked as though this was going to be somewhat of a challenge. I flexed my right arm in a show of strength but only succeeded in eliciting a face of scorn from Hayley. I put on my own serious face and opted for a change of position. I reasoned that I could get a little more force behind it if I approached the task from head on. As such, I knelt on the floor in front of Hayley and prepared to try again. After some more pea action we were ready and, as Hayley looked away for the third time, I finally pushed the needle into her. We were told to compress the syringe slowly but firmly, which I did but it was really tough to get the drug to pass into Hayley's body. It seemed like it took ages to empty and Hayley yelped for the first time in all the injections we had done.

So that was that. There was no going back now. The follicles that had been developed by the use of the Gonal-F injections over the past twelve days would very soon be getting a full dose of Ovitrelle. The Ovitrelle, basically, causes the eggs in the follicles to mature. In thirty-six hours time, Hayley's eggs should be ready for collection.

The next day we did precisely nothing except sit around watching television and singing random songs to try and encourage the eggs to finish with the growing and be released. It was a silly day and not one that I would care repeating too often. Although neither of us really said anything, there was an air of nervousness about the day. This was a big thing because tomorrow was harvest day.

The day arrives.

We had to be at the clinic by half past seven in the morning, so we had arranged to stay with Hayley's mother who lived a very short drive away. Although we were supposed to rest as much as possible we only managed fitful sleep at best. Hayley had to rest to make sure that the drugs worked as best they could and I had to make sure that my sperm were as good as they could be.

We arrived five minutes early and were immediately told by the nurse that we were twenty-five minutes late. We said that we were told to be here forty-five minutes before the collection and we were actually early. The nurse made mumblings about 7am, but did not push the point. Hayley and I simply looked at each other as if to say 'bit rude isn't it?' and then followed the nurse to our room. Now maybe I have watched too much television or read too many books but when I think of a private room in a private hospital, certain things spring to mind. I think of pristine Egyptian cotton sheets. I think of hardwood flooring and delicately patterned curtains. There is a flat screen TV on the wall and flowers on the antique table. What there was in actuality was a bed that looked like any NHS bed I had seen, with the slight difference that it went up and down by pushing a button instead of jumping on a foot lever. The bedside table was MDF with slight staining and the least said about the curtains the better. We were definitely not talking The Savoy here, more Bates Motel with a better cleaner. Still, it was at least clean and it did have a television. A television that only showed ITV, but a television nonetheless.

While I was mulling over the finer points of private hospital accommodation, the nurse got on with taking Hayley's blood pressure, before weighing her and asking her to wee in a pot. I did note that her wee-pot was smaller than the pot I got to use. Maybe they do it on purpose to stop the men getting cocky. Once the pot had been filled and taken away, our consultant put in an appearance and got Hayley to sign some consent forms, although she had no idea what she was consenting to as the handwriting was so appalling. She signed them anyway and the consultant went away saying that he would see her in theatre.

Hayley had just stolen the television remote, claiming she hated GMTV and surely there must be something else on, when a new person knocked and entered the room. We asked who he was and he said 'I am the anaesthetist' in much the same tone as you might say 'We are your firing squad'. There was a definite glint in his eye as he said it. Next was a quick trip through Hayley's medical history for the anaesthetist's benefit before he too announced that he would see Hayley in theatre and left the room. We had been at the hospital for about twenty minutes by this point and we were finally alone in our room to ponder the enormity of what we were about to do. The pondering lasted all of thirty-five seconds before the nurse blustered back in and declared that it was time for Hayley to go down for egg collection.

To recap. It was getting on for eight in the morning and I was sitting alone in the uncomfortable chair in a private fertility clinic room in Kent. My wife was in the operating theatre and I was watching a man with silly hair cook something wholly inappropriate for the hour of the morning. God, I needed sleep. There was now nothing that I could do about Hayley's side of the IVF. About now she would be going to sleep and soon the eggs would be extracted from her and placed in a dish. Nothing at all could change the quality or quantity of the harvested eggs. They were what they would be so there was no point in worrying about it. Something I felt was worth worrying about was that at some point in the reasonably near future I would have to 'perform' as the doctor had put it during our last meeting. By 'perform', of course, she meant to have a quick one off the wrist, a shifty Sherman, choke the chicken, scrub the bunny, fondle the fondue, or any other of the vast number of euphemisms that I could come up with. I had never had to give a sperm sample anywhere other than my own bathroom so I had no idea what to expect. I had visions of being led to a room without a name plaque (presumably because no one could think of what to call it) and being presented with some tatty porn from 1973. I imagine that the clinic would be professional enough to make sure that you don't bump into anyone else who is giving a sample that morning, but what if the chap before you is running late or can't sort himself out? Will I end up waiting in some adjoining room while he does his business, hoping not to make eye contact as he comes out of the 'W' room? Will the room be cleaned before I get to go in or will I have to take my chances with any spillages that may be waiting there? Another thing worrying me is how long do you spend in there? Do you go for the thirty seconds 'wham bam' type affair? It would be the best way of getting it over and done with but will you get withering looks and comments of 'I bet that has never happened before' and 'It's ok, you can try again in a couple of minutes' from the nurse, who I am presuming will accompany me to the room? Or, do you really take your time and settle in to it? Maybe have a seat and make yourself comfortable. Actually, given the amount of occupants that the room would have had, sitting down is possibly not the best idea. Okay, so standing up but still taking a little time and getting as relaxed as you can before you do the deed. You could ask the nurse to get you a cup of tea and maybe a custard cream. Hmm, maybe a different biscuit as it goes. Of course, you run the risk of losing track of time and spending too much time in your room. There could be several men all waiting outside, trying not to look at you as you leave, but all thinking you are a complete weirdo. What if there are several blokes, all running late, and you have to go in together, all clutching your own pots? Talking of the pot, what do you do with it afterwards? Do you hand it to the nurse so she can say well done? I bet she won't shake your hand though.

While I was sitting on my own having my introspective moment, Hayley was being taken down to the operating theatre. When she arrived, there were eight people already waiting in the theatre. Two were the anesthetist and his assistant; two were introduced as embryologists and neither of us have any idea at all who the other four were. After Hayley lay down, she had a drip inserted and they started giving her antibiotics. A few minutes later, they started pumping in the anesthetic and got on with the task in hand.

While Hayley was sleeping, a doctor would have been ex-tracting her eggs. We knew that she had around twenty-two good sized follicles, each of which may contain an egg. We had administered the big nasty injection to mature the eggs and so it should all be very straight forward from this point. The procedure itself is quite simple. The idea is that the doctor will push a very thin, hollow needle into the woman's vagina and then into each ovary in turn. One of the unidentified people in the operating theatre will operate the ultrasound scanner so that the doctor can see where he is sticking the needle. The needle is very obvious to see on the scan and the follicles appear as dark, round patches. Once the needle is in one of these dark patches, the fluid in the follicle is sucked down the needle and into a dish. The follicle is then completely drained and an embryologist takes the dish and its contents which are thoroughly examined under a microscope to see if there is an egg contained therein. This process is called follicle aspiration. Assuming that the embryologist finds a viable egg, the dish, egg and all the fluid are taken and placed in an incubator for safekeeping. This process will be repeated in its entirety for each and every follicle until all are drained.

We had been told that the embryologist would write the number of eggs found on Hayley's hand so that when she came around she would know exactly how things had gone. For some reason though, this did not happen and as she groggily opened her eyes as she was being wheeled into the recovery room the first thing she did was to look at her hands. When she saw nothing, she looked again, panicked and shouted for the nurse.

It was some time later when Hayley was wheeled back in to our room. I was still watching rubbish daytime TV and had not seen a single other person since Hayley was taken to theatre. She smiled as she was wheeled in.

'How many?' I asked.

'Fourteen,' she said, grinning from ear to ear.

It was a lovely moment to be able to share and I was glad that no one had come in and told me how many eggs we had before they brought Hayley back to the room. With Hayley's bed back where it should be, the nurse gave her some painkillers and said that she would be back to check on her in a little while. Although Hayley was excited about the number of eggs that we had, it did not help to take away the pain she was in, neither for that matter did the painkillers she had taken. We told the nurse, who came in with a little cup of oral morphine, which apparently tasted foul but did make Hayley a little more comfortable. Now Hayley was reasonably settled, I could get back to worrying about the impending sample I would have to give. I had still had nothing explained to me about the room I would be taken to or if there would be any reading material to help things along if you follow my drift.

Thankfully, I did not have too long to ponder such things for our embryologist, a chap called Steve, arrived and said that the time was here and it was my turn to provide him with what he needed. He handed me a plain folder and a pot and said that I could use the en suite to do what I needed to do. Steve left the room at this point, leaving me alone with Hayley and the pot. We looked at each other and Hayley raised an eyebrow.

I took up my pot and clasped the folder under my arm before giving Hayley a kiss and heading off into the bathroom. It was one of the weirdest feelings I have ever felt. Pretty much all men have popped to the bathroom for a quick Tommy Tank: many have clutched a certain type of magazine as they go. I personally had never done such a thing in a strange bathroom with my wife waiting outside the room knowing full well what I was up to behind closed doors. I locked the door because I did not want a nurse to walk in and although Hayley was sharing the whole experience with me, I did not feel that me wrestling the end of my willy so I can direct its flow into a pot was any sort of spectator sport.

I took a deep breath and wondered where to start. The first thing to do would be to relax I thought. Well, I may as well see what delights were in the folder. It was a single and rather tatty copy of a well-known top-shelf publication. It was one of the men's magazines that pretended that they were not soft porn, although they featured fully naked women. As part of the pretence of being taken seriously, the magazine featured articles and interviews. The interview in the magazine I had was with the punk bloke from *The Prodigy*. Now, call me Mr. Picky here but that just does not do it for me at all. I flicked through the rest of the magazine in the hope that something would get me all excited but to no avail. So, I quietly put it back in the folder and tried to think of something more suitable to the process. I have to say the mirror that covered one entire wall of the bathroom was not helping matters, but with a little cunning positioning and lots of happy thoughts, the pot was used and the deed was done. For reasons that I have yet to understand, Hayley said that she was proud of me as I emerged from the bathroom brandishing my pot. She even took the pot from me and whispered to its contents about being good and looking after her eggs. After a short wait, Steve appeared again and took the pot away to do what he needed to do with it, returning only briefly to collect the porn.

As Hayley and I left the hospital, our eggs and sperm were in the hands of Steve and the other embryologists. My sperm was evaluated then washed and spun to remove all the gunk. It was then evaluated again to make sure the planned course of treatment decided upon by our consultant was still applicable. I assume it was as the embryologist team went ahead with the ICSI. They took all fourteen of the eggs that had been collected from Hayley and put them all in separate dishes. Next, my sperm was studied under a microscope and one of the best, presumably one that looked like it knew what it was doing, was sucked up into a tiny needle and injected into the first egg. This process was repeated for the other thirteen eggs and all the dishes were left to culture over night. By this point there is nothing that anyone can do to aid fertilization. Quite simply, it will either work or it won't, so they are best left to get on with it.

We were told that we would get a phone call the next day between nine and ten in the morning to let us know how many had fertilized. We were also reminded that it was not impossible, although quite unlikely, for none of the eggs to fertilize correctly. The journey home was notable for three reasons. Firstly, it took absolutely ages as we had to keep stopping so that Hayley could stretch out and walk around for a while. Once the follicles had been drained, Hayley's body was determined to try and fill them back up with fluid as quickly as possible. The practical upshot of this was that she was feeling very bloated and uncomfortable. Secondly, Hayley was understandably feeling quite sore internally where the needle had made its way up through her insides. Sitting down was not the best position to be in. Finally, the egg collection would appear to have an unpleasant side effect that we were not aware of – wind. Copious amounts of wind. The handy thing about this was that I could use Hayley's wind to cover my own that appeared to be trying to compete for the whole duration of the journey.

Surprisingly, we both got a pretty good night's sleep that evening. I think Hayley was so tired after the collection and the anesthetic, nothing would have kept her awake. For my part I have the ability to not worry about things that I can do nothing about. I was well aware that I could not do a thing to help the eggs and sperm do what they needed to do so I was not going to worry about it. There was also the chance that the treatment would work and that at some point in the future, we would have a baby. If this were the case, then I was going to get as much sleep as I could when I could.

The next morning, we were both up early and spent the morning staring at the telephone, which was conspicuously not ringing at all. I even found myself picking it up periodically and checking that it still had the dialing tone. We drank far too much tea, we ate too much toast and we failed to distract ourselves from waiting for the phone to ring. It did ring once, at just gone half past nine but it was someone claiming they were called Graham who really wanted to service our gas appliances. I can't remember exactly what I said but I have a feeling it was not entirely complimentary and may possibly have called into question the marital status of his parents when he was born. Anyway, he soon went away and we got back to staring at the phone whilst drinking more and more tea. By the time it was half an hour past the latest time that Steve said he would call, we had both had enough and decided to make the call ourselves. We got through to the hospital, who called down to Steve who relayed a message back to us that he would call in a few minutes. By this time, Hayley was doing a very good impression of a nervous wreck. She was pacing the house, saying various things that all started with the word 'what if…'

'What if none have fertilized?'

'What if none of the eggs were good enough?'

'What if the sperm were really rubbish?'

To be honest, she had a point. What if any or all of these things were true? It was not entirely unreasonable to think that we had not been called because nobody wanted to be the one to give us the bad news. It was equally possibly that we had not been called because everyone who knew what was going on with our eggs and sperm were up to their necks in work and we had simply been forgotten about. Just as I was considering making yet more tea, the phone rang. We both looked at each other and Hayley picked the phone up.

It seems that we were both worrying about nothing as, according to Steve, out of the fourteen that we had yesterday, eleven were mature enough to be used for the ICSI process. Now I am not an embryologist so I have no idea how you measure an eggs maturity. Presumably you tell it a joke about periods and see if it laughs. Anyway, these eleven mature eggs were injected with my eleven best sperm and left overnight. Of these, seven actually fertilized and made it to today. How cool is that?

We now have seven little embryo's sitting in dishes at the clinic and an appointment tomorrow afternoon at three o'clock to have two of them put back in.

This is a very strange time in the whole process and the one that I think finally started to drive home what we were actually doing. In an incubator many miles away were seven little embryos that were, genetically speaking, half me. All seven of these had the potential to become my child. I say potential as there was still a long way to go. There was nothing to say that any of them would survive the night and absolutely no guarantee that if any of them did, that they would stick to Hayley's insides and develop further. It is an easy thing to do as a man, or at least easier than if you are a women, but I felt that I needed to define what I felt life was.

It could be argued that all seven of the embryos were alive and from a certain point of view that would be true. They are alive, but they could not continue to develop without being inside a womb, so for the purpose of my own sanity, I decided to class them as potential life. They were one step up from sperm or an egg, but still only potential. If I believed that all seven were alive then I don't think I would have been able to do what we needed to do tomorrow and that was to accept that the two best ones would be put back into Hayley and allowed the chance to develop and that some of them would probably be left to fade away. This is not as harsh as it sounds and should certainly not be something to put you off the idea of IVF. There is a lot of evidence to suggest, although no full research can ever be carried out, that many people get this far when they are trying, or not trying, for a baby the traditional way.

Getting pregnant is not quite as simple as the sperm finding the egg and managing to burrow its way in. Once this has happened, the fertilized egg will split into a two-cell embryo. It will then split into four cells, then eight and so on and so forth. As it is doing this, the embryo will move into the uterus and bury itself in the thick lining. That is if it all works of course. It is quite possible that the egg or the sperm may not be completely right and that the cell division will not happen correctly. It may be that the division is fine and that the embryo fails to lodge in the uterus lining. It may be that it lodges fine and then fails to develop and gets absorbed in the very lining it was meant to be safe in. Any of these things could happen and the woman it is happening to could know absolutely nothing about it. The scary thing is that no one has any idea just how often this is happening. So generally speaking, if you are going about baby-making in the traditional way, you do not know if it has worked or if it is in the process of working until the women concerned misses a period. I was in a position that many people are never in. I knew that I had seven potential children. They were miles away in a dish and, with any luck, they would be happily dividing their cells until tomorrow afternoon when they could be popped back where they belong. It was a very strange feeling indeed but, do you know what, I liked it.

Having said all that about defining life and potential children, I still failed to get any sleep that night as I was far too excited about the embryos. We were approaching the final stage of IVF and it had all worked so far. Having read several peoples' stories, I could not believe how lucky we were to have got even this far on our first attempt. There was a tiny part of my brain that kept trying to get my attention by saying that the luck had to run out at some point. I chose to ignore this tiny part and think about the seven little embryos growing in a dish all those miles away.

5. Embryo transfer

Having failed to listen to my own advice and therefore failed to get any sleep, I gave up with all things bed related and wandered to the kitchen to commence tea duties at about six in the morning. Hayley managed a little more sleep but the uncomfortable feeling in her insides kept her awake just as much as fretting about the embryos did. We pottered around for a while but failed to achieve anything useful and eventually headed off to the clinic. When we got there, we had to wait for a while but were eventually taken to a side room where we were met by the embryologist, Steve. He explained that of the seven embryos that we had yesterday, one had not developed very well at all, one was developing a little too fast and five were doing exactly what he would have expected them to do.

The idea with fertilized eggs is that they should double their amount of cells roughly every twenty-four hours. So a day after fertilization, the embryo should have two cells, four cells the next day and so on. Our embryos were now two days old and so should all have been four cells in size. The one that was developing too slowly was only at three cells and the one that was a little too far ahead of itself was at five cells. The worry for the slow developer would be that it might never catch up and the one going too quickly could just get out of sync with Hayley's body. All in all, Steve explained, it was easier to stick with the ones that were exactly on track.

It is worth pointing out at this stage that different clinics have different policies when it comes to transferring the embryos back into the mother. The clinic we were at had the policy of transferring on the second day after fertilisation. Some will wait until day three and some will let it go even further than that. If it were a traditional conception then the embryo would generally start to imbed into the lining of the uterus around six days after fertilisation. This is not set in stone by any means and it can happen a few days later. This is an important point as it is this imbedding that triggers the body to manufacture the pregnancy hormone known as human chorionic gonadotrophin (or H.C.G.), which is what pregnancy tests look for to give a positive result.

We were told that the embryologists would select the best two out of the five and those would be the ones that would be put back in Hayley. I have no idea what this selection process involved, but there are times when you just have to bow to other people's knowledge and experience.

We were led into the transfer room where we were met by our consultant, a nurse and Steve. The consultant told Hayley to remove her lower clothing and to lie down on the hospital bed that dominated the room. The nurse held up a towel for Hayley to hide behind as she attempted to remove her jeans. There was some giggling as taking her jeans off proved to be more than a little difficult as she was still suffering from a very sore stomach following the drugs and egg collection. However, they were soon removed and Hayley took her position on the bed. She had to lie so that her bottom was right on the edge of the bed and her feet were in the attached stirrups. This was easier said than done as the consultant kept on asking her to move down. After much shuffling, we were ready to begin. I say 'we' but my job was to sit by Hayley's head and keep quiet. I did have time to muse on the subject of fertility consultants and the odd view they must have on the world. With the exception of the occasional meeting, the most they see of people are when they are laying flat on their backs with their legs in the air. Sometimes they are even conscious. Thankfully, I was derailed from this thought process by the consultant asking the embryologist to get ready. Behind closed doors, our two selected embryos were put into a dish and sucked up into what looked like a pipette with a very long straw attached to it. The embryologist then checked the dish under a microscope to check that the embryos had definitely left the building and then passed the straw to the consultant who was positioned on a chair staring straight into Hayley's bits. The big light on the movable arm was then turned on so that he could see what he was doing and the speculum was inserted. A quick squeeze later and the straw was passed back to the embryologist so that he could check that it was empty. He disappeared back behind the scenes and emerged a short while later to say that the tube was empty and to give us a big grin. The consultant then said that we should stay here for while and relax. He wished us well and left us in the little room with only the nurse and our thoughts for company.

Unsurprisingly, Hayley shed a few tears at this point. Technically speaking, she was now pregnant with twins. As I said before, when you do IVF you are in a very privileged position insofar as you know that there are a certain amount of fertilized embryos in there whereas in traditional baby making you have no idea until much further on. The downside of this knowledge is that you know what you have to lose should it not work. There was not really anything we could do now, so we chatted about pointless things with the nurse until Hayley decided that she was as relaxed as she was going to get and it was time to be brave and attempt putting her jeans back on again.

6. The two week wait

This bit is most definitely the worst part of the whole process.

Once the embryos have been put back, you have to give them time to develop, to keep cell-doubling and to imbed themselves in the uterus lining where they will, if all goes well, grow into babies. The embryo would usually implant into the lining on around the sixth day after fertilisation which would trigger the release of the pregnancy hormone. By two weeks after fertilisation, you should be able to tell if the implantation has worked and if you are pregnant. However, two weeks is a bloody long time.

If you are going about the whole thing in the non-IVF way, then you may share a 'was that the one?' moment after sex, but you keep going on with life until something occurs to make you think that something may be happening on the baby front like a missed period. We found that carrying on as normal was only possible for some things. Firstly, Hayley was in far more pain than someone would be if they simply had sex to get this far. The follicles in her ovaries had now filled back up with fluid resulting in her stomach appearing very swollen. This means that she let out a little yelp every time she moved or bent over. Things are not really made any better by the next lot of drugs that Hayley had to take. The cyclogest pessaries had now arrived. The ones that we were told had to be inserted up your bits, one in the morning and one before bed, but could also be stuck up your rear end if you didn't fancy popping them in the front. Well, they are about an inch or so long and coated in wax, which is meant to make them easier to insert. This may be the case but it also means that you have half-melted wax leaking out of your bits most of the time. They are supposed to help thicken the womb lining and generally make your insides nice and sticky so that the embryos stick where they should do. This may be the case but they are pretty unpleasant for the person who has to insert them into themselves. You may say that if I was truly a modern man who really wanted to share in the whole IVF experience then I should of at least offered to do the inserting myself, especially since Hayley is not at her most flexible at the moment. I would like to state categorically that if this is the case, then I am not a modern man at all. There are limits to any relationship. One is that I refuse point blank to ever be in the situation where one of us is brushing our teeth while the other is on the toilet. The other is that I am not poking miniature candles up my beloved for anyone or anything. Sorry, but there it is.

Moving on, the internet is a wonderful thing. However, it can also send your lady slightly mental during the two week wait. There are all manner of websites and discussion forums that offer advice and huge lists of things that you should and should not do while you are waiting to find out if your little embryos are going to stick or not. Luckily, Hayley took much of the advice with a very large pinch of salt. We both decided that a healthy diet was probably a good idea and Hayley continued cutting down on caffeine, so we now had two boxes of teabags in the cupboard yet again. The fridge was suddenly filled with fresh vegetables, the ice cream supply was not being replenished and the fruit bowl was taking on a life of its own. Gone were the week old bananas and in their place were pineapples – lots and lots of pineapples.

Every morning Hayley now took her folic acid pills, her iron supplements and her vitamins before having a cup of decaffeinated tea and a whole pineapple. This is after she has cleaned up the wax and inserted a new candle of course. She then tried to take it easy as much as possible as everyone we spoke to agreed that the worst thing you can have is stress. The other things to avoid are, apparently, being too hot, being too cold, chemicals, heavy lifting, ironing, climbing ladders and having sex. Some of these things were not as easy as they sounded and some were very easy. Hayley had no issues whatsoever with avoiding heavy lifting and chemicals. She reasoned that most of the chemicals that she could come into contact with would be the ones used for cleaning and, as such, had drafted her mother in to deal with that. I felt I had had a rather lucky escape but decided that keeping quiet about it was probably the best idea. The only time that Hayley was likely to climb a ladder would be to go into the loft and that was never going to happen. In our house, as in many others, the loft is the man's territory. Avoiding being too hot or too cold was a little trickier though as there were still an awful lot of hormones trundling around Hayley's body from the injections. The practical upshot of this was that she had started to have hot flushes. They could happen at any time of the day or night and there was not much she could do about them. Of course, the night ones were worse from my point of view as they would involve her pushing the duvet off as hard as she could. The duvet would then end up doubled over and all on top of me. I would then half wake up, push the duvet off and go back to sleep. Once the hot flush had passed, Hayley would then wake up because she was too cold, realise that the duvet was nowhere to be seen and wake me up to go and retrieve it. The no sex rule was actually one of the easy ones to keep. Firstly, Hayley was not feeling even slightly sexy what with the pains and the swelling and the fact she had bits full of wax for most of the day. Combine this with the fact that the constant fighting over the duvet was not leading to a amorous bedroom atmosphere, we managed to keep our hands off each other with minimal fuss. The final thing Hayley was told to avoid was ironing. As far as I was aware, the ironing board was still in the plastic wrapping that it came in several years ago so this was not going to be an issue.

The things that people were saying that Hayley should do were things like take light exercise, go for walks, sleeping, relaxing, keep positive and avoid stress. It was the last one that was to cause us a problem but more of that later.

As we continued our wait, Hayley's tummy continued to grow and then her nipples changed colour. Without any warning, tea suddenly made her feel sick. This may have been the foulness that is caffeine free tea but maybe not. It seemed that every time I popped back into the house from work, she was eating boiled eggs. Okay, sometimes she was munching on one of the many pineapples that we had in the house, but mainly it was eggs. It was possible these symptoms could be down to her period being due, but a little part of myself was still allowing me to believe that maybe, just maybe, they were signs of early pregnancy.

We did encounter a few issues with the whole idea of avoiding stress. Well, the *idea* of avoiding stress was perfectly fine; it was the actuality of doing so that was causing us issues. For example, we were meant to be going down to London for a screening of a film that I had worked on. This had the potential to be a stressful experience but with the aid of cabs and a little care and attention, we reasoned we should be fine. However, on the morning of the day we were due to go, we got a call saying that Hayley's grandfather was very ill and had to be rushed to hospital. We dashed to the London hospital that he was in but as he had to be taken straight into surgery there was really nothing we could do. The doctor later told us that Hayley's grandfather would be very ill afterwards and in intensive care for quite a while. It would appear that no one bothered to tell granddad about this as he was awake within a couple of hours of leaving theatre and half an hour after that was demanding his dinner. Hayley's stress levels were raised to say the least!

On day three of our wait, Hayley emerged from the bathroom carrying a pregnancy test. We were told very firmly and specifically by everyone at the clinic that we should not do a test until the fourteenth day. The fertility drugs would give silly results and could possibly cause false hope if we tested too soon. It would appear that Hayley had selective hearing during that part of the discussion. Her reasoning was thus:

The fertility drugs in her system could cause a fake positive result on a home pregnancy test. If we were lucky enough for one or both embryos to implant, then Hayley's body would start producing its own pregnancy hormone at some point after day six. So the only way that she would know for sure if the reading on the test was caused by being pregnant or by the fertility drugs was to do a test very early on and then another a bit later to see the results go from positive to negative as the fertility drugs cleared her system and then, hopefully, back to positive as the pregnancy hormone built up after implantation. Today's test showed a dark blue 'pregnant' line. Hayley placed the test in a drawer and continued with her day as if this was perfectly normal behaviour.

By the end of the first week of our wait, things were still looking good. Hayley had continued doing pregnancy tests daily, sometimes even twice. They had started out as 'positive' but the little blue line had got fainter day by day until today it told us that Hayley was not pregnant. Oddly, we both classed this as good news. It meant that the hormones caused by the fertility drugs had now reduced to such a level that they could not be detected by the little stick that you have to wee on. This meant that if the little blue line appeared again, it would definitely be good news. Could it be too much to hope that somewhere inside Hayley's uterus, one or both of the tiny embryos could be attaching themselves to the lining and developing into a foetus? Personally, I felt that it was still too early to start hoping for such things.

We had some other good news today too: it would seem that Hayley's swelling had gone down slightly. Not enough for her to be able to wear her normal trousers so she was still living in her track suit, but it definitely seemed to make things a little easier for her. Her breasts were not hurting as much as they had been either. Now if I was a negative person, I could read into this that things were not happening down below, but her period had still not arrived and the moods that tended to arrive the week before the bleeding had also not happened. Admittedly, Hayley was still not able to drink tea and her consumption of eggs was continuing unabated, so things were certainly not back to normal by any degree.

Within a couple of days, Hayley's bloating was back with a vengeance and both of us were finding it really hard to concentrate on anything at all. On the plus side though, the Sky planner was no longer full of baby programmes. I had still failed to watch the episode of *Top Gear* that I had been trying to watch for weeks, but you can't have everything, can you? In order to distract ourselves, we ploughed through the DVD box set of a well-known anti-terrorist drama that is set in real time.

I also realised that there are two smells in this world that I absolutely cannot stand. One is coffee and the other is cooked egg. Given that Hayley was off tea at the moment and craving eggs pretty much all the time, the kitchen was not a pleasant place to be for me. At the end of the first week of waiting, the pregnancy test showed a very faint positive line. There was a chance that this could be some left over hormone created by the treatment so we did not get excited about it. Well, maybe a little.

As we trundled along through the second week of the wait, Hayley was still disappearing into the bathroom clutching a little stick to wee on. We were only doing the cheap own-brand ones, mainly because we did not want the cost of the pregnancy tests to eclipse the cost of the IVF. Every day the little blue line was getting thicker and thicker. Still neither of us could believe that this little blue line would stay and would mean that Hayley was with child. We were still at the point where most people do not know if they are pregnant. It was not quite two weeks since the sperm and egg met so it was very early days indeed. Even if the tests were right and one or both of our embryos had managed to lodge themselves in the lining of the uterus, there were still a lot of things that could go wrong. Given Hayley's history of two ectopic pregnancies, the most immediate concern was that one of the little chaps had not lodged in the correct place and had somehow managed to drift up into what remained of her fallopian tubes. If this was the case, the pregnancy test would still give a positive result but could lead to a very bad situation. Basically, if we had another ectopic, then there was a chance that the doctors would have to remove Hayley's womb, making it impossible for us to have children. The clinic specified that we must wait two full weeks before testing so we could not call them at this point because all they would say is that we tested too early and to call back on the day they told us to test in the first place.

As we neared the end of the two-week wait, we encountered a problem. Hayley's swollen tummy was now making it impossible, rather than just awkward, to put on her jeans and she was point blank refusing to continue living in her tracksuit. We assumed this was nothing to worry about but called the clinic anyway. They said that it was probably just the fluid filled follicles and that unless the pain got worse it was not worth getting checked out. That was all very well but she could not go through life wearing the grey tracksuit bottoms that were currently the only thing in her wardrobe that fitted. Admittedly, we could have moved to certain areas of south-east London where the wearing of such items was classed as essential, but we figured the easiest thing to do was to go shopping for something else for Hayley to wear. I did offer to find some tracksuit trousers myself to wear on our shopping trip but I was told not to be sarcastic.

We went off to the shops, both glad of something to concentrate on that was nothing to do with sticky insides and imbedding embryos. Unfortunately, if you go up a size in jeans, they assume that all of you is bigger and not just your stomach. We rapidly found that the only clothing option we had was to be found in the maternity section. Now herein lies a problem, well several problems actually. Firstly, Hayley was not keen on wearing maternity clothes when she was not yet officially pregnant. Secondly, would wearing them mean that we were taking a positive result for granted and tempt fate? There was also the feeling that if it did not work then we would have these maternity clothes in the house when no one was pregnant and that was a little odd.

I pointed out that it was a very old fashioned view that only pregnant people could wear maternity clothing and that the forward thinking person should be able to think of several situations where they would be handy. You could keep a pair of maternity trousers handy to wear on a Sunday afternoon after a particularly belly-busting roast dinner and avoid that whole top button-loosening scenario. The over-bump trousers could be very handy on cold days where you want a little extra warmth over your tummy but not necessarily all the way up to you neck and the tops could be worn to disguise some rather unsightly trapped wind. I think Hayley thought that I was talking rubbish, but it at least made her laugh enough to stop worrying about wearing maternity clothes at this time. So, we bought a single pair of jeans. I had to admit that buying too many things might be tempting fate just a little, and Hayley popped to the toilets to change so she could wear them home.

It was a Friday. It was test day. Even though we had now spent the equivalent of a small country's national debt on pregnancy tests, all of which had been giving a positive result for the last few days, I was still convinced that today, when it mattered, the test was going to be negative. Unlike when we started the whole process, where we had the camera out and the tea on stand-by, there was no ceremony this time. Unless you count the hurried opening of the posh, and therefore expensive, pregnancy test box. With the box duly opened, Hayley went off to the toilet to wee on a digital stick. According to the blurb that came with the test, it could take up to three minutes to register a positive result. It didn't though. It took about ten seconds to reveal just one word:

PREGNANT

'Bloody hell,' I exclaimed.

Hayley simply nodded, gave me a hug and shed a silent tear.

I made tea before we phoned the clinic of course. They were obviously pleased and booked us in for a scan in two weeks time, with a note to the effect that we should report anything out of the ordinary, such as bleeding or spotting in early pregnancy and if Hayley had any pain at all then she should go and see her doctor.

Once off the phone, Hayley began making a list of all the people we had to tell. With traditional conception, it is the done thing to wait until you are twelve weeks pregnant before making any kind of announcement. With IVF, it is often the case that close friends and family know what you are doing, so as soon as the waiting is over they all want to know the result. Whilst Hayley was doing this, I took the time to just sit and try to work out how I was feeling about the situation.

It was the pregnancy test that had me puzzled, not the result, for that was spelt out in front of me. I, however, puzzled about my own feelings. As we had been progressing through our treatment we had many little goals. Firstly, we had the goal of lowering Hayley's FSH, then we were trying to make follicles and then making those follicles larger. We then had to aim for a good amount of eggs followed by a decent amount of sperm that had a clue where they were going and were able to get there. The next goal was to get as many eggs fertilised as possible and finally for the embryos to stick to Hayley's insides. This was all very distracting and now that we could say that we had officially been successful at IVF, I came to the realisation of what this actually meant.

It meant that Hayley was properly pregnant. I know that sounds really silly, but I was so wrapped up in the whole IVF process that the end result seemed to have slipped my mind. There was another person growing inside my wife, possibly another two people. All those people we had watched on television, going for scans and going through labour, would soon be us. There is a further stage to this as well: in nine months time I was going to be a Dad. That is something I was going to think about a great deal, as soon as it sunk in that Hayley was pregnant. Walk before you can run and all that. First things first, we had to deal with the clothing issue. One pair of maternity trousers was just not going to cut it, so it was off to the shops for us. Living the dream? Oh yes!

Ruby Thursday Rebecca Saunders
was born on the 3rd July 2008 at 14:08
by natural delivery, weighing 5lb 15oz.

7. Frozen embryo transfer (FET)

When we had our first full cycle of IVF, we had managed to get five little embryos. Two of these were popped back in, leaving three left over. These were shoved in a freezer for use later on. I say freezer, but it is not the same as the household appliance you would use to keep your ice cubes in. Well you might, but it would be a bit odd.

Whereas IVF is not, by any means, a precise science, has an awful lot of variables and relies on a certain amount of luck, embryo freezing has to be bang-on accurate. Whilst many people refer to having embryos in the freezer or fridge, it is nothing like that at all.

The theory of being able to freeze living things and thaw them out so that they are still alive has been around for many years. Someone worked out a long time ago that there must be a temperature that is as cold as you can possibly get, maybe after a wintry night out in Leeds. This temperature has been theorised to be several different things over the years, but the current consensus of the scientific community is that it is -273.15 degrees centigrade, and this is known as Absolute Zero. The theory goes that this is the temperature where all molecular movement stops. If you keep something at this temperature it should remain exactly as it was and never age. As you warm it up again, the molecules should start moving and carry on from where they left off before you chilled it. There are one or two slight flaws with this in practice though. The first one is that it is not actually possible to create a temperature that low, but we can make things pretty cold if we put our minds to it. The second issue is that all living cells contain water, which has the alarming habit of turning to ice as it gets cold and even a tiny ice crystal can damage a cell if it is poking into it. Even if you can get whatever it is you want to freeze cold enough and are lucky enough that there are no sharp bits of ice sticking into it, there is then no guarantee that it will survive the thawing process.

Back in the forties, a team of scientists were trying to work out the best way of freezing bird sperm for later use. There may have been a good reason for this but it may just have been a distracting hobby. Due to a labelling mishap, one test tube, containing wildfowl sperm, was filled with the wrong chemical. This chemical was called glycerol and had the lovely effect of working far better than anything they had tried before. What they were trying to find was a chemical that would prevent the build up of the potentially damaging ice crystals, and, completely by accident, they did just that.

So, after many more years of research and a fair amount of trial and error, the scientific community arrived where we are today. As far as IVF goes, the cryogenics are reasonably straight-forward. Once you have an embryo that you wish to keep for later on, it is placed into a series of complicated solutions in order to draw out as much of the water from the cells as possible. Once this has been done, the embryo is placed in a cryoprotectant chemical very similar to the one discovered by accident all those years ago in order to protect it during the freezing process. It is then cooled slowly over about three hours until it is at minus thirty-six degrees centigrade. At this point, the embryo and its container are plunged into liquid nitrogen where it remains until it is needed again. The liquid nitrogen keeps the embryo at minus one hundred and ninety-six degrees centigrade. Although this means that there is still some small molecular movement, the embryo thawing process from this temperature is far less likely to involve complications or damage to the embryo than if it was frozen at a lower level.

All that is what happened to our three remaining embry-os. They were frozen on the second day after fertilisation and were both four cells in size. They had been in the freezer for over a year when Hayley and I decided that it was about time that we had a conversation about them. Most storage facilities charge by the year so we figured we should probably talk about things before we got an invoice for another year's storage. Once we learned that Hayley was properly pregnant with Ruby, I pretty much put all thoughts of frozen embryos from my mind. It is not that I did not care about them; more that I had far too many things in my head and life at that time. However, the impending arrival of another bill sharpened my mind a little. We did what was fast becoming a tradition with all fertility related decisions and sat down with a nice cup of tea to work out what we were going to do.

If you have frozen embryos there are basically three things that you can do with them. Firstly, you can have them defrosted and leave them to perish, which, if left outside the womb, they will do fairly rapidly. Secondly, you can have them put back into your wife or partner to see if they grow and turn into babies. Thirdly, you can donate them.

The choices you make are in part governed by how you feel towards your embryos. Some people think of them no differently than they would do a child, others see them as merely a cluster of cells. Whatever you think though, they do have the potential to give you a child so the choices you make should be carefully thought out.

My feelings towards them were a little mixed. Whereas I did not consider them to be children, I was aware that given the right circumstances and a certain degree of luck, they could become so. I think I have some kind of in-built safety mechanism that stops me becoming emotionally attached to them. As far as I was concerned, they were not children; they were just the potential for children. If the conditions were right inside Hayley and if luck was on our side, then they could grow into babies, but at the moment they were not. I think Hayley felt more attachment to them than I did, but it would be her that would have to carry them for nine months if we put them back and they stuck, so I could understand this completely. That said, I know people who are as attached to their embryos as I am to our daughter, so there is no wrong or right feeling towards them.

So, tea made, we had the conversation that we had been putting off. Although we both knew we were going to have a go at having them put back in at some stage, we thought it only right to go over all the options. We both decided that the option of letting them perish was not, in fact, an option. It was not that we felt they were alive, just that they could be in time. Having them stuck back in again would mean more cost, more drugs and more worry so we moved on to the third option for the time being.

There are two ways of donating unwanted embryos. Firstly, you can donate them to medical research and secondly, you can give them to another couple who can have them put in and hopefully get pregnant. From my point of view, both of these options have good and bad points. The idea of donating our embryos for medical research was something that I felt strongly against. There were all sorts of great reasons to do this. They could be used to improve fertility treatments, maybe reduce the risk of miscarrying and any number of potentially fantastic things. Unfortunately, the people who donate the embryos have no way of knowing what research they will be involved in. The logical part of my brain was telling me that all research into fertility must be a good thing as there are so many people out there who cannot conceive and the medical profession have no clue as to why. The part of my brain that has watched far too much television over the years was conjuring up images of evil geniuses in laboratories in hollowed out volcanoes, conducting research on the cells that could have been my children. Okay, so I had no evidence to back that up, but the thought was there and something in me had decided that while I was all for people doing research into fertility issues, if I was going to be involved, or at least my genetic information was going to be involved, then I wanted to know what they were going to be doing with it.

The other donation option was even more of a moral minefield. If we chose to donate our little cell clusters to another couple we could, potentially, be giving them the greatest gift they would ever get: the chance to carry a baby and have children. Part of me really liked that idea. However, it is not that simple, certainly not in the UK anyway. It is not as simple as meeting a couple, thinking they are nice and wanting to help them out. If you donate, then you have no say in the couple that get your embryos. They could go to anyone, even people who, if you met them in the street, you would not like. This is obviously a problem because although I did not consider the clusters of cells in the fridge to be my children, if they developed into fully formed babies, then they would be half me and then I would definitely say that they were mine, genetically anyway. Did I want to have my children being dragged up by some unwashed chav? Probably not. Again, this was the illogical side of my brain talking. The sensible side of me was thinking that if you were at the stage where you have no choice but to use donated embryos then you would have tried everything else and would be getting pretty desperate for a child. The people who received the embryos would have to have private treatment, as the NHS does not do it, so they may be reasonably well off. Not that your relative wealth has anything to do with your parenting ability of course. But the fact that recipients of either eggs or embryos have to be pretty well off does mean that you should not have to worry about your DNA becoming a child who has to want for the material things in life. They may still be left wanting for the emotional things, but that is something that is unrealistic to speculate about. Look at it like this and it was not such a bad idea.

The thing that stopped me wanting to donate to another couple was the fact that Hayley and I had a child already. Although the embryos were half me and half Hayley, they would be 100% genetic siblings to our daughter. As the law currently stands, neither Hayley, I, or our children are allowed to know where the donated embryos went. Should those embryos turn into babies and subsequently children and adults, they *are* allowed to know about us. All of us, including their genetic siblings. My personal feeling is that this is not fair on our daughter and I was not prepared to do something that could result in her having a brother or sister that she is not legally allowed to know anything about unless they come looking for her first.

Having discounted the options of disposal or donation, we were left with two choices: either pay for another year's storage or pop them back in and see what happened. Many people say that there is never a good time to have your first child insofar as you will never have enough space, time or money. The same can definitely be said for your second with the added fun that you have to take the age of your first into consideration. If there is only a year or so between them then they will have things in common and hopefully be able to play with each other. The downside is that you could end up with two or more children under two years of age, which could certainly be far more than a handful. If you decide to wait a bit longer, then the older one will be less trouble when there is a tiny baby around and may even help to look after the little one as they get older, but the two of them will have less in common the larger the age gap between them is. We figured the best course of action would be to have a go and see what happened.

Once we had decided, Hayley called and made an appointment with the same consultant that we had seen last time. We thought it was worth a chat with him just to see what was involved, how much it was all going to cost and what the waiting time was. We got an appointment the next week. In the week between the conversation and the consultant appointment, I had completely failed to think about our embryos in any way at all. You could say that I was not taking this seriously, but we had a one year old to look after and a business to run so there was not really a lot of time for embryo related introspection.

The day arrived and so did we, at the clinic that is. Having taken our seats, realised that the chairs were still in need of some industrial beige remover and found that the gossip magazines were now even more out of date than the last time we sat here, we were called into the consultant's office only ten minutes later than our appointment time.

Our consultant said that frozen embryo transfer or FET was generally simpler than a full cycle of IVF. There were two ways of doing it. One was a medicated cycle whereby Hayley would have to take pretty much the same drugs as she did before in order to get her insides prepared to receive the embryos. The other and far simpler option was a non-medicated cycle where her natural cycle would be used and the embryos returned at the appropriate point. We explained that Hayley's cycles were generally thirty days but sometimes slightly more. Our consultant said that this should be good enough and said that there was a free appointment to see the nurse in a couple of weeks.

Twenty minutes later we left the clinic having made an appointment to see the nurse and start our second IVF journey. Neither of us was particularly sure how that had happened.

'I thought we were just going to talk about it,' I said.

Hayley made 'hmm-ing' noises, agreed and we went back to our lives. I tried to work out how I was feeling as we drove home and came to the conclusion that it had not sunk in at all yet. It was all very well saying that we were going to go and see the nurse and get some more drugs of course, but we had so long to think about our first cycle that this seemed a bit fast. Still, I reasoned, the clinic must know what they are doing. I had failed to put much more thought into the whole thing by the time we turned up to see the nurse two weeks later. It was not as exciting as our first time I have to say, in fact, I got the distinct impression that the clinic considered an FET to be a little beneath them. There was no sense of excitement and no great 'this is it' moment. The meeting was purely informational and we left having been tasked to pick up another big Ovitrelle injection and some more pessaries, although no one mentioned the other hole you can stick them in this time.

'So are we really doing this?' I asked.

'Well it seems so,' was Hayley's response.

Neither of us could quite believe how quickly we had been signed up for an FET. When we had been thinking about starting our first IVF cycle, we had read up on it, spoken to people who had done it and found out everything we could to help our chances. We still had a box of caffeine free tea in the cupboard that we were both stubbornly refusing to drink. We had studied statistics and googled consultants. Hayley had been to the funny women with the needles and I had taken a variety of vitamin pills and fretted about masturbation. This time though, neither of us had done any preparation at all and yet we were pressing ahead. We had a little while to wait as Hayley was not due to start her period for a while, but once that was over and done, we would be checking to see when her body was ovulating and then off we go.

As I said before we had both done nothing to prepare for the FET. Now this may be because we had a one year old to look after or it may be that neither of us really thought that it was going to work anyway. At the clinic we were using success rates for frozen transfers were quite a lot lower than those for a full IVF cycle, but they did work and there was no reason for either of us to think that this one would not. For me, the whole thing felt different to last time. It may have been the lack of build up or the fact that I did not have to change anything about my life but it just did not feel as though we were doing anything special. Life carried on as it had been doing until Hayley's period arrived. Again, there was no pomp or fanfares just a quick phone call to the clinic to say that it had come and what did they want us to do now?

The answer was not much. We had been told that Hayley should ovulate somewhere between days fourteen and eighteen of her cycle, so we had to go for an ovary scan on day fourteen just to see what was going on in there and to make sure that Hayley was producing a dominant follicle and that the lining of her uterus was thickening up nicely.

I can remember during our first cycle that there was a lot of waiting around and doing not very much at all. Although there was not quite as much this time, we managed to fill the wait quite easily with chasing after the baby and not thinking about IVF. Every now and again I would glance at the calendar and see that the date of the scan was approaching and still I felt no excitement, trepidation or anything much of anything. There really was nothing to do, no changes to make in our lifestyle and no pot to use or abuse. I felt redundant, useless and pointless all at once. Don't get me wrong here, if it worked then I would be excited. I would leap around and make whooping noises, but that voice in the back of my head, the voice that only had good things to say during our first treatment, that voice was saying that there was no point getting excited about things as it was not going to work and the best thing that could be said for the whole thing is that it gets me away from work for a day or two while we have the scans.

It is incredibly difficult, although not technically impossible, to have your embryos moved from the hospital or clinic where they are stored. They are yours so you can choose to take them somewhere else for further treatment but it is not as simple as popping them in the post and waiting for them to turn up. The equipment used is very specialized and therefore very expensive. I say this as in between having our embryos frozen and deciding to have them thawed and put back in again, we had moved house. We now lived just over one hundred miles away from the clinic.

The morning of the first scan arrived and we set off when it was still dark. By the time the sun was grudgingly making its way into view, we were half way down the motorway and nearing our destination. We staggered, bleary eyed, into the clinic and announced our presence. We were soon met by a doctor and taken to one of the ultrasound rooms. The scans at this stage were of the internal variety so it was a case of pants off, feet together and legs apart. For Hayley at least. I just sat on the uncomfortable chair and waited for some information to come my way. The doctor appeared happy with what she saw and said that Hayley's ovaries were progressing nicely and could we please come back the day after tomorrow.

On balance, what we should have said was something along the lines of 'it takes three hours to get here and you insist on making us have early morning appointments so we have to get up when its dark and drive a long bloody way and no I don't want to do it again'.

What we actually said was, 'Of course. See you then.'

Spineless, the pair of us.

So we drove back home and spent another couple of days going about our business and not really talking about the impending transfer. I still don't think that either of us wanted to admit how unexciting the whole process was.

We had the next scan two days after the first and all was still going well. According to the doctor Hayley should be naturally ovulating in the next two days. Two days time was a Saturday so we were asked to come back the next morning. Neither of us really wanted to do the hundred mile drive again the next day so the doctor said that we could do a home ovulation test that should tell her everything that she needed to know.

I was so relieved that we did not have to drive down two days on the trot that I failed to think of the thing I thought of once we got home. The issue was that when we were doing our first full cycle, Hayley was taking fertility drugs and being scanned until she was almost glowing. This time around we had two scans and were now putting the future of our embryos plus the thousand or so pounds we were being charged on a home ovulation test that I had absolutely no faith in. My lack of faith was on the grounds that if these home ovulation tests were 100% accurate then everyone would be using them and we would have a far greater population problem than we currently do. However, I figured the doctor must know what she was talking about so we put the test in the bedroom and had a spot of dinner.

If we had been going through a medicated FET, then things would have been very different. Hayley would have been taking some of the same drugs that she did for our full cycle and, I presume, her insides would have been monitored just as vigilantly. As it was though, we were at home on the day that our clinic suggested was the most likely day for Hayley to be ovulating, with nothing to pin our hopes on other than a small stick. A small stick that Hayley took to the bathroom and promptly had a wee upon. She emerged a couple of minutes later, still with the stick in her hand, which was then placed hygienically upon a piece of kitchen roll on the table. The instructions said that the result could take up to five minutes to appear so we stood in anticipation. After only a minute or so the control line and the positive line both appeared. We played it cool though and waited the full five minutes just in case one or both of the lines decided to disappear again. Luckily they did not so we could be reasonably sure that the test was right and Hayley was indeed ovulating.

You would have thought that this would have been cause for celebration, and that we would have been straight on the phone to the doctor to tell her the good news. Instead of jubilation, the over-riding emotion was just a sense of 'Oh? Are we? Right you are then.'

We called the hospital after a while and let them know. The doctor seemed quite happy for us and said that everything was all very good and that we would be having the embryos put back in Hayley on Tuesday afternoon. Of course it would not be as simple as that, or at least may not be. With all things in IVF, nothing is a given and that is definitely true for a frozen embryo transfer. As Hayley sat on the phone and I stood a few feet away trying to work out what was being said, our three embryos were in a controlled environment with the temperature fixed at one hundred and ninety six degrees below zero. Or, to put it another way, pretty bloody cold. Although there were all kinds of safeguards and protection measures in place, there was absolutely no guarantee that any of the embryos would survive the thawing process. The process itself is quite simple and basically involves getting them out of the fridge and letting them warm up by themselves until they get to room temperature. The embryos are then dunked into four separate solutions to remove all of the chemicals that were used in the freezing process. Finally, they are warmed up to body temperature and mixed with a little solution to give them something to float about in while they are waiting to be placed in a uterus. There is a fair chance that the embryos will come out of the process undamaged, but many do lose at least one cell and if you only had four-cell embryos to start with, like we did, you could encounter a problem. The thawing process is timed so that they are in the solution for as little time as possible before being put back into the uterus. This meant that no one would be able to tell us how many of ours had survived until about two hours before transfer when we would be somewhere on a motorway. Still, as an anonymous wise man once said, 'If you are not living life on the edge, you are taking up too much space.'

Hayley thanked the doctor and put the phone down. She filled me in on what was said and reminded me that she also had to start taking the cyclogest pessaries again to make sure that the lining of her womb was nice and thick, all ready to accept any embryos that may have survived the freezing and thawing processes. But before we could start on the lovely little wax tubes, we had to do the big injection. The ovitrelle injection was the same one that we had to do during our first cycle. Again it came with a worryingly thick and long needle that required the injector to take a run up in order to get enough power behind it to actually get the damn thing to go in. All the way through our first cycle, there was a little voice in the back of my mind saying that I should not worry as it will all work out okay in the end, and despite several occasions when Hayley was determined it has gone wrong, I had this little voice and something inside me knew that it would be fine. I still had that little voice now. The problem was that it was not telling me that everything was going to be fine. It was telling me I should not worry as it would be pointless to worry about something that was destined never to work.

That night we actually sat down and spoke about what was going on. We both felt that there was nothing special about the whole process. I elected not to mention the little voice of pessimism in my head, but we both felt that there was not the same air of gravitas from the clinic staff this time around. There was not the same feeling from us either now we finally came to talk about it. We knew that the success rates for FET were lower than for a fresh cycle and the fact that ours were frozen as two day old, four cell embryos meant that the chances of them thawing were not the best and the likelihood of them implanting once thawed were even less. Even though we knew this, we both felt that we could not progress on to a second fresh cycle while we still had embryos on ice. They would always be there, eating away at us, making us wonder 'what if?' The best way of making sure that we could get on with our lives, we felt, was to give it a go and see what happened. The worse case was that it would not work and then we could start looking into a fresh cycle again. The best case is that it does work and then all the pessimism would have been a waste of time and we would instead need to work out what to do with two, or maybe three, kids.

As Monday arrived, I felt a bit odd to be getting on with work while a hundred miles away three little embryos that could each become a child were being taken out of frozen storage and left to thaw. Admittedly there was nothing I could do if I were there. In fact, there was nothing that anyone could do other than to monitor their temperature and make sure that no one dropped them on the floor or anything like that. The three little chappies were now on their own for a day. All they had to do was warm up and then we could see how much damage the freezing process had done to them. Every time we stopped for tea, which given our track record was quite a lot, we ended up speculating how they were doing and what temperature they should be at by now. Our anthropomorphic embryo fantasy came to an end that evening though when reality barged in and demanded that the pessaries be dealt with. Hayley left it until bedtime before trudging off and doing what needed to be done. Strangely, neither of us felt the urge to reminisce about all the pessary related fun we had last time around. I fell asleep, failing completely to feel any trepidation regarding tomorrow's transfer.

Hayley did not sleep as well as I did, although the timid voice of Ruby demanding 'milky' in the small hours of the morning did briefly interrupt my slumber. As we bumbled through our morning routine and made sure that we had arrangements in place for the rest of the day regarding Ruby and work, we still had no idea what was happening with our embryos. We were still non-the-wiser as we got into the car and headed off on the hundred mile journey.

The phone rang as I was attempting to use the force of my mind to persuade an Audi driver that he did not want to insert himself into my rear end. Hayley answered it as I turned the radio down. There was a lot of nodding and umm-ing noises from her as the Audi finally got the message and pulled into the outside lane, presumably figuring that there was far more success to be had in the concept of 'around' rather than 'over' or 'through' that they had been trying previously.

Hayley flipped the phone closed and let out a sigh. She then explained that all of our embryos had now been thawed but none had survived unscathed from their freezing experience. When they went into the fridge they had all been four cells in size. Now we had one that had degraded down to two cells and two that had lost one cell so were now three cells in size. The embryologist said that there was no point at all in attempting to put back the one that had halved in size and it would be best to let it perish and concentrate on the two larger ones. As Hayley and I had very limited experience in fertility matters at that point, we accepted his word as gospel and continued on our journey.

The conversation for the rest of the way down to the clinic mainly consisted of speculation regarding the likelihood of a three-cell embryo doing what it should do. There are many reasons why a frozen cycle may not work. One is that the embryo does not continue to grow following the degradation caused by the freezing and thawing processes. The other is that the chemicals and hormones in the female body are just not quite right for the embryo to stick where it should. I mention these two, as these are things that no one has any control over at all. The embryologists will do all they can and modern science is pretty clever when to comes to cryogenics, but if the embryo has been damaged, then it may not continue its growth. There is also the possibility that the embryo in question would have started to fail on day three of its life anyway, whether it had been frozen or not.

As we neared our destination, we both decided that the conversation we were having was doing nothing to put us in the right frame of mind for embryo transfer, so we tuned the radio to a phone-in station and amused ourselves by laughing at the people ringing in.

Our consultant greeted us as we entered the clinic's reception area. He led us down a corridor and into the same room that we had been in when we had our previous two embryos put back over a year ago. It was the same drill as last time with Hayley doing much bottom shuffling until the consultant was happy that both Hayley and himself were in the correct position. He then asked us some questions to make sure that we were who we said we were before the embryologist arrived brandishing the floppy syringe that held our two thawed and slightly reduced embryos. I toyed with the idea of mentioning that it may have been more pleasant for Hayley if the questions had been asked before she was positioned into the stirrups, but by the time I had thought of something suitably pithy to say about it, the consultant had already squirted the contents of the syringe into Hayley's insides and was in the process of handing back the vessel to the embryologist, who took it away to check that it was completely empty and that they embryos were definitely inside Hayley. Once everyone concerned was happy, Hayley was allowed to remove her legs from the stirrups, the consultant said his goodbyes, wished us luck and left us in the little room with only a nurse and the embryologist for company. We thought that this would be the time to have a chat about the freezing process in a little more depth, which killed enough time for the nurse to be happy that we could go on our way. As we were about to leave, a thought occurred to us. We asked if it would be possible to have the dish that our embryos had been in before they were squirted back into

Hayley. Although we had failed to ask for the dish that contained Ruby, we thought that, whatever the result of the transfer, it would be nice to have the dish as it would be nice to explain to all our children how they came about. Apparently, we were the first people at the clinic to ever request this but neither the nurse nor the embryologist could think of a reason not to comply with our request. They even found us a bag to take it home in.

We popped the dish into Hayley's handbag, said our goodbyes and left the clinic for what would be the last time. We wandered to a nearby garden centre for a spot of lunch and took a leisurely drive back home. From a certain point of view, Hayley was now pregnant with twins once again, or at least she had two little fertilized embryos floating around inside her. We were now into our second two-week wait, although hopefully this one would not cost us quite so much in pregnancy tests.

It was a very different feeling this time around. The anxiety that we both felt last time was replaced with something close to frustration. The more we thought about it, the more both of us felt the treatment wasn't going to work. We were both very worried about the lack of care we felt we received at the clinic this time around, which was a marked difference to the first IVF cycle. It was as important as ever that Hayley tried to get a much rest as possible, which allowed her to spend a reasonable amount of time on the internet researching the FET protocols for other clinics. What we discovered was that embryos that had been frozen on the second day after fertilisation were very unlikely to take once they had been returned to the uterus. I am not a great believer in statistics but it seems logical to assume that an embryo that only started off as four cells in size and then shrank down to three would stand less chance of working than one that was bigger to start with.

After a few days, Hayley popped off into the bathroom to pee on a stick just to see what was going on. The result was a resounding negative, which was what we had expected. We now knew that all the injected tomfoolery was out of her system and so if we did get a positive result in the future then it was a proper positive and not some hormone left over from the ovitrelle.

The anxiety continued on my part well into the second week of the wait. I had pretty much convinced myself that nothing was going to happen and started to feel angry about it. I was not angry that Hayley was not going to become pregnant. There are so many people out there who have many goes at IVF and never get a baby, so the fact that we were lucky enough to get a successful outcome on our first attempt made me feel that I had no right to get grumpy if the FET did not work. It was not the idea of a failed cycle that was annoying me: it was the way the clinic had gone about it. The thing that I really did not understand was that when we were doing our first cycle and were waiting to see if our eggs and sperm could get it together in a fertilising sense, we were told by the clinic that any embryo that was under four cells in size by day two would not be good enough to be put back in. However, the clinic was more than happy to put into Hayley two thawed out embryos that were less than four cells in size. The cynic in me was thinking that if they had been a little more consistent with their reasoning then we may well have got a phone call to say that none of our embryos had survived the freezing process and it was best to abandon the cycle. However, if that had been the case then the clinic would not have been able to charge us an extortionate amount of money for the transfer.

As I said, this may be an overly cynical point of view, but it is very hard to be objective when everything that you read is telling you that the embryos inside your wife are not going to work, that you are not going to be a father again, at least not this time. After the first week of our waiting, we decided that reading things on the internet was not as good an idea as we had previously thought it to be, in fact we stopped completely. Hayley didn't even do many pregnancy tests either. She did one or two of course, but nowhere near the amount that she got through during our first two-week wait.

During our first wait, we were completely focused on the treatment in hand, we religiously studied pregnancy tests and, as we got closer to test day, finally allowed ourselves to speculate on what life would be like if the treatment worked. This time around though, I think I stopped thinking about the impending result at least four days before that result was due. So much so that Hayley and I found ourselves talking about our next treatment, which would have to be another full cycle and trying to work out when and if we could afford it. The store card affair that we had taken out to pay for our first cycle was still pretty full so there was no way we were going to be able to use that for another go. We decided not to get ahead of ourselves. Just because we both felt this cycle was not going to work did not mean that we were right and we still had a couple of days until the official test day so the best thing to do was nothing until we knew for sure what was going on inside Hayley.

The answer came on test day at around ten in the morning. We had one of the posh digital tests that did not simply give you a number of little blue lines, but instead told you in plain English whether you were pregnant or not. I had always wondered what the point of this was, as if you could not figure out the difference between one little blue line and two then you probably would not be able to read and almost definitely should not be breeding. However, the fact was that we had one of these wonderfully technically advanced little gizmos, so Hayley wandered into the bathroom and took a wee on it.

The result came through quite quickly again, the words fading into view as we sat on the sofa looking at the test:

NOT PREGNANT

Well, that was that then. Put the stick down and step away from the pregnancy test. Nothing to see here, move along, move along. I shrugged and flicked through a couple of television channels to see what was going on. For some reason I always have to be doing something else in order to think about the thing that I should be thinking about in the first place. As I flicked through some obscure and high numbered channels, my brain started to digest the information. Not pregnant. Right … well … hmm … although it had not exactly come as a surprise, it was still not pleasant news. Although I had a feeling that the FET would not work, I guess I must have still had a little hope in me somewhere because now I knew that we were not going to have more children, I really wanted them. Maybe it is that thing when people tend to want what they cannot have. Whatever the reason though, I was now determined that we would find away to have more children. Unfortunately I had no idea how we would go about it. I should say though that I simply felt that we had had a failed treatment and not that we had lost a baby. Different people have different ideas about what constitutes life. For me, embryos are only a potential for life. This may be right or it may well be wrong, but I do not think I could handle a failed treatment if I believed that the embryos were our children.

Of course, Hayley did not take it the same way as I did. Although she knew that the result was not going to be positive, it still hit her pretty hard when the final results came in. Even though she was convinced that it was not going to work there was still a little voice of optimism whispering from the shadows of her psyche. Hugs and tea were the order of the day.

Some people believe that fate plays a large part in life and love and all things. Myself, I am undecided on this matter but all I do know is if there is such a thing as fate then it has a warped sense of humour because three days after we had called the clinic to tell them that the treatment had not worked, fate, or whatever you may call it, conspired to kick me squarely in my underperforming balls. My fathered died and succeeded in taking my mind completely off the failed treatment.

8. Full cycle with egg share

It was almost a year after our failed frozen embryo transfer that we started another journey on the road to Babytown. As we were still paying for Ruby, there was no way we could afford to pay for a full cycle again, especially as the health authority we were now under had closed the loophole that allowed us to get our drugs paid for the first time around. Clearly we needed a plan.

When we had been going through our first full cycle, Hayley had found an article on the internet about something called 'egg share'. It was a story about a couple who had tried pretty much every kind of fertility treatment that there was including several goes at full IVF. After years of trying, the doctors had finally concluded that the reason for the lack of success may well be because the woman's eggs were not strong enough. The only option left to the couple, apart from adoption, was to use another woman's eggs. The man would still be the biological father, but the woman would not be the biological mother if the treatment worked. I found it fairly amazing that the treatment actually worked and they had a baby. When you start to look, there are hundreds if not thousands of people in similar situations; people that go through heartache after heartache and thousands and thousands of pounds only to get nothing at the end of it. All they want in life is to have a child of their own, to carry and give birth to a new life, to look into the eyes of a newborn and be able to say 'we did that'. For many of these people, the only option they have is to use donor eggs and in some cases donor eggs and donor sperm or even a complete donor embryo. As we read about the couple who had a baby through donor eggs, we decided that if we got a baby from our first go then we would both like to help a couple who were not as lucky as we were by donating some of Hayley's eggs. This was far more Hayley's choice than mine as they are her eggs to give away, but the idea of being able to help another couple have a child was something that really appealed to both of us. That had to be the most wonderful gift that an infertile couple could receive, didn't it? I say gift, but the more we looked into it, we more we found that it was a gift the recipient most definitely had to pay for.

There are only a handful of clinics that do egg share and they are constantly advertising for donors. In addition to this, the current laws in the United Kingdom state you cannot donate your eggs for money. In other countries the people who are going to receive your eggs will pay you to undergo the egg production stages of IVF as well as cover your expenses and things of that nature. You then hand the eggs over, take your expenses and leave them to it. There is no such thing in the UK though. Firstly, the clinics who take donated eggs prefer that you have no contact with the person who is going to receive your eggs and you are not involved in the process of choosing the recipient. They could go to absolutely anyone at all and you have no say in it whatsoever. So if you have a problem with your eggs going to someone that you deem unsuitable, then donating eggs is probably not for you. The thing is though, you have to be very well off to use donated eggs because not only do you have to pay for your own IVF cycle, but you have to pay for the people whose eggs you will be receiving to have a full cycle too. When you combine this with the fact that the clinics that offer the service do not tend to be the cheapest out there, then you will be looking at a bill well in excess of ten thousand pounds. As I said before, having money does not mean that someone will be a good parent, but it does mean that we would not be helping someone create yet another child born into poverty. We did talk briefly about what kind of parents we would like Hayley's eggs to go to, but we soon realised that madness lay down that road. We could have speculated forever about what the people would be like, what kind of demographic they would most likely come from in order to be able to afford the treatment and what kind of short-comings would be traditionally associated with that sort of person. However, it is completely impossible to tell if anyone will be a good parent until they try. The thing we did take solace in was that anyone who was prepared to undergo not only IVF but IVF with someone else's eggs, would most definitely want the resulting child more than anything else in the world and if you want something that badly, then surely you will look after it as though it is the most precious thing in the whole world.

There are moral issues with egg donation as well as financial ones. From the woman's point of view any children born will comprise fifty percent of her. There is also the fact that those children can find out who donated the egg they were made from when they get older, so there is a chance that one or more children might turn up and want to be part of your life at some point in the future. There is also the question of what happens if you run out of eggs and can't have any more children but you donated eggs to other people that you could have used? At the end of the day, it is something that both of you have to be completely comfortable with and definitely not something to be entered into lightly. Hayley and I talked about it, on and off, for nearly a year before we saw a post someone had left on an internet forum. This person was looking for someone to sign up to be an egg donor at a London fertility clinic. Although we had not met the woman who posted the message, we both thought that it would be a nice thing for us to help her.

This was not entirely the selfless thing that it could have been; it was also a case of economics. We could not afford to pay for another full cycle and the fact we now had a child meant that we were no longer eligible for a go on the NHS. If we agreed to donate half of the eggs that Hayley produced under stimulation, the person who got the eggs would get the bill for our treatment, which if we went to the same clinic as the lady whose internet posting we had read, would be around seven thousand pounds just for our bit.

It is not an easy decision to make though. Well, it is from a male point of view because it would not be my eggs that would be donated. I can certainly see how Hayley and many women would be very attached to their eggs, after all they only have a finite amount of them and generally only have access to one every month. Men, on the other hand, generally have as much sperm as they need and often show no restraint in spreading it far and wide. Hayley bounced between loving and hating the idea of donating eggs and every time we got a chance to talk about it, it seemed as though she had changed her opinion on the subject yet again. However, we had decided that if we were going to have another go at getting pregnant then it would have to be soon as we did not want the age gap to be too large between our children, assuming, of course, that the treatment worked. Realistically, the only way we were going to afford another go was if we got a very large loan or if somebody else paid. We were still paying for our first two treatments so getting more credit that way was not going to be possible and given the lack of eccentric millionaires kicking around Cambridge waiting to hand over wads of cash for fertility treatment, the second option was not looking too likely either.

We finally reached enough of a decision to make a phone call and arrange a meeting with the egg donation department of the clinic in London that the woman on the internet was at. The idea was that we would trek down to London and meet the egg donation nurses and a counsellor to talk about whatever it is that such people talk about and finally one of the fertility doctors. That way we could ask any and all questions that we needed to and they could go through all the stuff they needed to do, which was basically to work out if we were suitable for the donation programme or a pair of unbalanced lunatics. Sounded quite simple really. The clinic sent us a huge amount of paperwork straight away, which we dutifully sat down and read as soon as it arrived. We then spent almost an entire evening filling out the very long and detailed forms that accompanied the reading material. We faxed them off to the clinic first thing the next morning.

We now had a few weeks to wait until our appointment and Hayley continued to change her mind on a daily basis mainly because she had been emailing the woman who was looking for donors and sometimes felt that the woman was trying to pressurise her into signing up for the programme. By the time the day of the meeting came around, she was feeling quite positive about the idea, focusing on the good thing that we would be doing for a couple that neither of us knew yet. By this time we also knew Hayley's eggs would not be used for the woman who had put us onto the idea in the first place, as she had just started treatment at another clinic with a different egg donor.

After a very dull train journey we arrived in London and took a stroll along the river from the station to the clinic. I have to say that this was much more what I was originally expecting from a private fertility clinic. It was a large, imposing four storey building that overlooked the River Thames. My brain was already fantasising about the lack of beige that I hoped would grace the insides as we walked up the steps into the reception. It appeared that this hospital had a number of departments as the middle aged man on reception, who had looked almost pleased to see us when we walked in, looked down and mumbled as soon as we mentioned fertility. We translated a particularly monosyllabic grunt as 'please go to the left and take the lift to the second floor' and did as we were told. We wandered down a chrome and hardwood walkway and into the fertility clinic. The décor was looking good so far so we walked up to the fertility reception desk.

There we waited. And waited. And for good measure waited some more.

As society and technology has progressed, we have made machines that can measure time down to a fraction of a fraction of a millionth of a second. None of these machines would have been fast enough to measure the amount of time that the women behind the reception desk looked up from her computer screen to signal that we should tell her why we were there before returning her gaze to whatever it was that she had been doing before.

We said who we were which caused a few seconds of frantic button pushing on the part of the woman who then nodded to herself and said that we should wait in the waiting room. She may have looked up again at this point, but if she did then I missed it. After glancing around the reception area, we spotted a doorway that lead into a room that was full of people sitting around and looking bored. Recognising the standard waiting room template, we made our way inside and found two seats. They were not next to each other, of course, as everyone in the room was doing their best not to sit next to anyone else, so each couple were their own little island, separated from the rest of the room by an empty chair on each side of them. Hayley and I were forced to plonk ourselves down in two of these separating chairs and sit there in silence. After about an hour, enough people had vacated their seats to allow us to move and sit next to each other, which we did just as one of the grumpy people from reception came in to tell us that we had not sent the forms in. We patiently explained that we had faxed them through weeks ago. The woman went away, presumably to look again for our paperwork, but returned shortly afterwards with some blank forms and told us to fill them out. As the first set had taken us over an hour to complete, we were not best pleased at having to do it all again. As it happened though, we had an hour to kill before anyone turned up again whereupon they asked me to follow them.

I was lead down a corridor with thoroughly dull art gracing the walls and shown into a little room. The room contained a suspiciously wipe-clean sofa, what looked like a bedside cabinet and a tiny door, about six inches high, set into the wall in the far corner. I was presented with a pot and told to pop it through the tiny door and ring the bell once I was done. I was not told as much, but I figured they wanted a sperm sample. Resisting the urge to sit on the sofa and have a nap, I went instead to look in the cabinet. Here I discovered a pile of porn that would have the average teenage boy holed up in his bedroom for at least a month. Thankfully there was not an article on punk rock techno bands anywhere to be seen. I did what needed to be done, popped the pot where I was told and rang the bell. After that, it was a short stroll back to the waiting room, trying to avoid eye contact with anyone else in there (as I presumed they all had a fair idea where I had been and what I had been doing), to take my seat back next to Hayley that she had thoughtfully covered in coats and bags to deter anyone else sitting there.

I sat. We waited. Another hour passed and finally some-one called both our names and asked us to follow them to an office.

We both sat down in the office feeling a little grumpy due to the three hour wait to actually get seen by anyone. Then a nurse came in and we started to go through all the things that the clinic would have known had they not lost the extensive form we had taken the best part of an evening to fill in and fax to them. We explained why we needed IVF to conceive and how our first cycle and subsequent frozen embryo transfer went. We also explained that the reason we had come to talk about egg donation was because of the woman on the internet. The nurse made dour nodding motions and explained that we looked like very good candidates. We were told that there were a few more things we had to do before we could officially start the process. We had to see a doctor, which we were scheduled to do today and a counsellor, which we would do after seeing the doctor so that we could talk about any issues, fears or neurosis we had. After that, Hayley had to go and have blood tests to make sure she did not have anything nasty. We then had to wait twelve weeks before having the same tests again to make sure we had not picked anything up in the meantime. Neither of us was inclined to think of any questions for the nurse, mainly because she gave the impression that she was far too busy and disinterested to answer them in the first place. So, with that being well and truly that, we were herded back into the waiting area to find we had to sit apart yet again as everyone continued their quest to not talk to or even sit near a stranger.

After another hour trying to lip read the news channel that was on the far-too-small and silent television in the corner of the waiting room, we were called by another nurse and told that the doctor would see us now. The doctor was unique insofar as he was the first person I saw smiling. Whether he had just heard a particularly funny joke, I do not know but at least he was friendly. That was where the usefulness stopped, as he did not tell us anything that we did not already know. I think the clinic thought we would need the whole IVF process explaining. We did not, so the meeting with the doctor was a little pointless. He told us the counsellor would call for us as soon as she was ready.

There was a small problem with this though in that the counsellor had gone home. Did anyone think to tell us this as we sat in the waiting room once again? Did anyone think maybe they should check what we were doing in there? No and no. The way we found out was when we went to reception to enquire how long it would be and were told that as we did not have an appointment as there was no one there to have the appointment with. I tried to ask whether they realised we lived a very long way away and did they really think it was polite to ask us to travel all the way down here again for the appointment when it was their fault we did not have a counsellor to see. The answer appeared to be a blank look and more tapping on a computer keyboard followed by being told we could come back next week.

As we walked back to the station I was, to say the least, fuming. We had spent a grand total of thirty minutes actually speaking to people and over four hours sitting around waiting. I shall say that again. Four bloody hours, sitting around waiting. They had lost our forms, given us no information and expected us to travel all that way again purely because they were about as organised as a two year old. At that point I was ready to walk away and never go back except possibly to give them an invoice for the amount of my time they had wasted. What was the point though? They would probably lose it.

By the time our appointment to see the counsellor had arrived, I had calmed down enough to go so we made our way slowly and expensively down to London yet again. This time around I was not as impressed with the décor as I knew about the wall of grumpiness that would greet us once we got inside. Hayley was keeping far more positive than I, saying that they may have been having a bad day last time and that I should keep an open mind. I found it highly unlikely that nearly every single person that we met was having a bad day but I was here now so I may as well enter into things with a positive outlook.

An hour sat in the waiting room without any information as to when something may occur served to knacker any happy thoughts I had managed to muster. So it was with a heavy heart and a fair amount of huffing that I trudged into the counsellor's room. We were all introduced and had a little small talk before we got down to the nitty gritty of egg donation. The main point of the meeting was to make sure we both understood all the ramifications of donating eggs. We knew the donation was anonymous and we would not know anything about where the eggs went. However, we did find out that Hayley would be matched as far as was possible to the lady who receiving the eggs. Things like height, build, race, hair colour and the like would all be matched as closely as possible presumably so the recipient would not have to answer any awkward questions from people who did not know she had used someone else's eggs should her treatment be successful. We also had the option, which the clinic encouraged, to write as much about Hayley as we cared to. Things like her career, hopes, dreams, other children and anything that we felt might be of use to someone when they found out they had a biological mother they had never met. The information regarding Hayley's name, address and all this additional information would be kept on file and given to the child of the recipient once they were old enough and should they wish to know. Whilst we gave all this personal information, we were not entitled to know anything about the recipient or the possibly resulting child apart from one thing. One year from the date of egg collection, we could call the clinic and they would tell us if our donor eggs worked or not. That was it. If it had worked then we had to be prepared for someone to appear out of the blue claiming to be Hayley's child. We would have no legal obligation whatsoever should this occur so we were not likely to get stung for eighteen years worth of back dated pocket money, but we could well get eighteen years of repressed emotion and angst. This was something that Hayley and I had talked about and so did not come as a shock. We signed the forms and were told we would be contacted with the date of our next appointment once we had done our first set of blood tests.

We left the clinic having avoided the waiting room for a second time and wandered back to the station. On the way back though we got a phone call from the clinic saying that they had forgotten that Hayley needed to have a swab to check for a couple of nasty things that may be lurking inside her. With a fair amount of mumbling, we turned around and headed back to the clinic wondering again how on earth they were ever going to make us a baby when they were completely unable to organise the proverbial in a brewery. It also appeared that our excitement at having avoided the waiting room again was a little premature as we were lead straight back in to sit upon the uncomfortable chairs. Luckily, it was not too long and within half an hour Hayley was lead away to be checked for chlamydia and gonorrhoea.

The next week was very confusing. I still really liked the idea of helping someone else have a shot at having a baby, even though it was not going to be the person who we originally thought we were going to be helping. But I was not sure at all about the clinic. My reasoning was that if they could not make and keep simple appointments, could not give you any information when you were there and could not manage to have a set of forms without losing them, then how the hell were they likely to be able to do all the things involved in a full round of IVF? Hayley came up with a very good idea. She reminded me that the people who sit and sneer at the front desk are not the ones who do the treatment and we should not judge a clinic by its administration staff. The same principle that you should not judge a book by its cover I guess. She thought we should go ahead and have our HIV test and wait to see if they did actually call us with our next appointment. If both things went okay then we may get to meet the people that do the IVF bit and then we could make a decision about whether we trusted them or not. This seemed like a good idea and the last time we went to have a HIV test it was a bit of a laugh, so why not?

We were now playing the waiting game yet again. Hayley had her first batch of blood tests back at the clinic as our doctors would not do them. I elected not to go with her this time, partly because it was a long way, partly because the train fare was not cheap but mostly because I was trying to keep positive about the whole thing. I also had a feeling that another encounter with the dour-faced grump-monsters on reception would well and truly bugger up any positivity I had managed to muster. We now had to sit around on our bottoms for twelve weeks until we could go and have our final blood tests. Most of this time was spent deliberating whether we wanted to carry on with the clinic or tell them to go and do something rude to themselves. Personally, I had all the issues I have mentioned regarding their inability to make and keep to appointments but there was something else that was bugging me. I was of the impression that what we were potentially doing was pretty amazing, certainly for the people who would get our eggs, well Hayley's eggs anyway. What we were doing could well give a couple the chance to have a baby that they would otherwise not be able to have. So why were we not being treated at least nicely, with a smile? I am not saying that the clinic should have put bunting out and had a bunch of people playing trumpets upon our arrival, but possibly acknowledging that what we were doing was a 'good thing' would have been nice.

As with most things in life that I find annoying, it faded in time. By the time we had to call the GUM clinic and arrange to go in to have our tests done, we had both come around to the idea that we should give the clinic one more chance to redeem itself. We had done a fair amount of research on the place and most people had nothing but glowing praise for the doctors and embryologists. On the basis that we had met only one doctor, the only person who smiled at us in all the time we had spent there, and had met no one from the embryology department yet, we decided to go with the theory that the clinic used all available people skills on the medical staff and there were none left over for the front of house mob.

It was a different GUM clinic than we went to last time, but they were just as helpful and had no issues whatsoever with giving us all the tests we needed for the clinic. I managed to avoid an examination for the second time in my life and we headed home, ready to make the call to book our first proper appointment.

This time around the person we spoke to at the clinic seemed at least vaguely enthusiastic about us coming in to see them. We had to go back down to London again in ten days time for our paperwork and drugs chat. The chipper nature of the person on the phone went some way to alleviating the negativity I had been feeling towards them and I managed to keep positive for the whole ten days while we waited.

It was asking too much for me to keep it up during the journey of course. The trip into London was as pleasant as it was likely to be but once we travelled across the city, we both felt we needed a shower as we emerged from the tube station and made our way to the clinic.

Here, something amazing happened. The nurse who was meant to be meeting us was already waiting in reception and took us straight through to her room. The first point of order was to go through the paperwork. We had to sign to say that we understood the whole process and she briefly went over the law regarding egg donation again. We then got onto the issue that we may end up with more embryos than we could use and I had to sign a bit of paper to say what I wanted to happen to them should I suffer some freak and tragic accident. I said that as I would be dead, I doubted that I would care very much so I signed to say that I was more than happy for Hayley to use our embryos after my death should she wish to do so.

We went over the drugs again. Some of them were the same as the ones we had used before. The nasal spray was the same, as was the final maturing shot. The stimulating drug that the clinic decided to use was called Menopur and although it was designed to do the same job as the Gonal-F that we had used before it went about it slightly differently and the way of getting it into Hayley was different. The easy to use pen arrangement that we had on our first go was replaced with a syringe and two little bottles. We would have to take the first bottle that contained a liquid and mix in a little of the powder from bottle number two. We would then have to attach the needle to the syringe, pierce the top of the bottle we had used to mix the powder and liquid and suck up the correct amount of the drug before stabbing it gently into Hayley. We also had the big maturing injection to do before egg collection and then it was the lovely little waxy things that had to be inserted up Hayley. As I said before, I was more than happy to do the stabbing side of things but I really did not want to get involved with the insertion.

Next the doctor produced a sheet of paper and looked at me. I guessed it was time for the results from the sperm jury to come in. We were told pretty much the same as during our first treatment. I had lots of little swimmers, many of which were not moving very much and of those that were, few were going in the right direction. I was tempted to say they were probably bored with the amount of time they were expected to sit in the waiting room before being called into action, but I did not think that would get us anywhere so I made the kind of face that I hoped would say something along the lines of 'Oh well, sorry, but it's not the end of the world, is it?'

The difference between the results I had for our first treatment was that this time they were on the borderline between being recommended for standard IVF or ICSI. This meant that if we could get my sperm just a little better then we would not have to have the ICSI treatment. Although our recipient was paying for our IVF treatment, they would not be paying for the ICSI if we needed it and as we were now in London and London prices applied, that was going to be a scary amount of money.

Once all was done, we were given our own needle bin again and presented with a prescription to take to the chemist so we could get all our drugs, which were definitely being paid for by our recipient. The only thing we did have to pay for was the HFEA registration fee (Human Fertilisation and Embryology Authority). We put that on plastic, collected our posh needle bin and made our way back home to collect the drugs and wait for the start of Hayley's next period.

We went home via the shops as Hayley said that she had a plan involving my sperm. This is the sort of statement that would generally get my interest going but I failed to see how anything fun was likely to be achieved in the medicine section of the supermarket. Hayley picked up what looked like far more supplements and vitamins than we had during our first cycle and announced that I would be taking these on a daily basis until the day of egg collection and my next meeting with my pot. Her argument was that a few pounds spent now on things like zinc and vitamins could possibly save us a vast sum of money if they improved my sperm enough to not need ICSI. I could not find fault with this so I trotted home and got myself used to the idea that I would almost definitely rattle whenever I walked for the next two months.

For those that are interested, the cocktail of pills and supplements that Hayley had found for me consisted of zinc tablets as well as vitamins A, C and E. I also had a multi-vitamin pill for good measure. The science behind it is that the zinc should increase the volume of sperm that you have while the vitamins C and D should improve the overall production along with the motility of the sperm. The vitamin A has nothing to do with sperm production or quality at all but does have antioxidant properties and, according to the box the pills came in, can also help me see in the dark. I think Hayley's theory with the vitamin A and the multi-vitamins, was something along the lines of 'why the hell not'.

I have to say that from my point of view the second time around was certainly less stressful than the first full cycle we did. Although there was still the same amount of waiting around and hoping that Hayley's insides would do their thing a little faster, the anxiety was definitely less than before. It may have had something to do with the toddler charging around the house but I like to think that I was a far more relaxed person than I was before. Self-delusion is a wonderful thing, isn't it?

We also had the distraction of trying to explain to an eighteen-month old girl that Mummy and Daddy were going to have a go at having a baby. This was not the easiest thing in the world to do as her attention was generally held for ten seconds or the time it took to find something to stick in her mouth, whichever was less. By the time Hayley called the clinic to say that her period had arrived and we had been given a start date of the first day of her next period I was taking everything in my stride. Well I say that, but I think it was more a case of being emotionally retarded to the whole thing. Something in my head was not letting me feel very much at all about the process. Having had one cycle that I had a feeling was going to work and a frozen transfer that I knew would not, I failed to feel very much at all about the cycle we were about to launch into. I think it was partly because I had rather a lot going on with work and Ruby but mostly because I knew it was our last go for the foreseeable future. There was no realistic way that we were going to have the cash just kicking around to pay for another go until Ruby was quite a bit older, which then gave us the issue of a large age gap between the kids if it did work.

Being a bloke, I found that the best way to tackle this potential emotional bombshell was to ignore it and concentrate on something else. I was still suffering from a staggering lack of excitement when the time came to start the down-reg drugs. These were the ones that Hayley squirted up her nose in order to stop her reproductive system doing anything and were exactly the same ones we had last time. We soon got into the swing of it though: one squirt in the morning and one in the evening. As Hayley's body took all the hormones on board, she started to get grumpy again, which given she was basically going through the menopause in two weeks was hardly surprising. I handled the grumpiness in a very manly way yet again. I hid in the office and only ventured out when the shouting had stopped.

Soon though, we started the scary injection drugs. Unlike the synarel nasal spray that we had a fair amount of experience with, these were very different to last time. The drug was called menopur and came in two parts that had to be mixed together and slurped up into a separate syringe. The only plus side that I could see to using the syringes rather than the pens we had before, was that I could hold them up to the light and flick the ends in the manner much favoured by medical professionals in television dramas. This time around we elected not to document the occasion with photographs mainly because neither of us know how to work the timer on the camera and manually pressing the button whilst attempting to handle a needle does not sound like the best idea in the world.

After Hayley had the first few injections, it was time to go back down to London to get scanned. It was good news and there were several follicles all growing away nicely. The clinic said these scans were to assess follicle growth and for them to be able to monitor whether the drug dosage should be changed. As it happened though, the doctor was more than happy with the way things were going. The nice thing about the drugs that produce the follicles is that they tend to calm down the person taking them. The down-regulation drugs tend to remove a lot of the 'happy' hormones and these drugs start to replace them. So Hayley was getting happier and the follicles were getting bigger and more plentiful.

We had been told we had a number of choices regarding donating our eggs. We need a minimum of eight decent eggs in order to share them. This means that the recipient will get a minimum of four good eggs. If we get more than eight then they are divided equally between us and the person who is paying the bill. The eggs will be rated and we will get the top rated with the recipient getting the second best. We get the third and they then get the fourth and so on until the eggs run out. If we get less than eight eggs then we have a choice: we can either choose to give the whole lot to the recipient, which means that although our cycle will go no further, the lady who needs them will be able to get on with it. If we choose this option, then we will get another full cycle to ourselves at no extra cost. The final option if we have less than eight eggs is to keep them all for ourselves, possibly making evil cackling noises and carry on with our treatment. The big downside of this is we will get the bill. Not just the bill from egg collection onwards, but the whole thing including the bits we have already had. We both hoped that this would not become an issue as, if last time was anything to go by, we should get a good amount of eggs. Last time, we got fourteen so with any luck we would get a similar amount this time.

The day before we were due to take the final scary egg-maturing injection, Hayley went back down to London for the final scan. The news was that she had fourteen follicles, but we had no way of knowing how many of these contained an actual egg. On our first cycle we had twenty-two follicles, fourteen of which contained viable eggs. So if Hayley followed suit, we could be looking at eight or nine good eggs.

The next evening we got the scary injection prepared. The injection was really no scarier than any other but from my point of view it was a little intimidating as I knew from last time it took a fair amount of pressure to get it in and I was keen to show Hayley that I had remembered this and had adjusted the force of stabbing accordingly. The other thing is that it injects quite a bit deeper than the ones we had been doing so it was going to take longer to get the drug in and therefore be more uncomfortable for Hayley. It was the administering of this final injection that started to bring home to me what we were doing. As I have often said, at length to many people, I tend to find statistics generally complete rubbish. Clinics put out figures of how many successes they have had with various fertility treat-ments but no one really knows what chance you have at IVF until you try. Working on this theory, Hayley and I had a 100% success rate at a full cycle and a 100% failure rate at frozen transfers. As this was a full cycle again, then it could be argued that it was going to work. This was not true, of course, but when your brain is going into panic mode, logic is not something it often bothers with. What if it worked? How on earth were we going to cope with another child? What if it worked really well and we had another two? What if it was three or four or more?

The day of egg collection came around quite quickly. Hayley still had fourteen follicles and I had worked my way through our entire stock of sperm building supplements. We were as ready as we would ever be. It was now almost thirty-six hours since we had done the final and potentially bouncy injection to mature up the eggs Hayley had, so we hauled ourselves out of bed at some thoroughly unpleasant hour of the morning and got in the car. We had found a car park that was not too far away from the hospital as Hayley did not want to fight her way through the middle of London and then sit on a train all the way back having just had a needle poked into her ovaries. After a brief struggle trying to get the pay and display machine to work, we arrived at the clinic just as the morning sun was poking above the London skyline. I felt that things were definitely looking up as the reception staff were not yet in and we were met by a nurse who, instead of leaving us in the waiting room that time forgot, showed us up to a ward. Actually the word 'ward' does not do it justice. There were only two beds in it for a start and these were quite far apart and separated by some not-too-unpleasant curtains. Each bed had its own private bathroom with nice, clean fluffy towels and a selection of designer toiletries. The view out across the river was fantastic, although it was easy to get distracted by the flat-screen television, and the tea was not too bad at all. Not that Hayley got any tea as she was not allowed but as all I had to do today was to get intimate with my pot, I made with the tea drinking with much gusto. In exchange for having no tea, Hayley did at least get a comfortable bed to lie down on while we waited for her to be called to the operating theatre. I got a chair that initially looked as though it would be a nice place to sit but was angled in such a way that as soon as you relaxed you started to slide down. Had I attempted to get a little shut-eye, then I am sure I would have woken as I fell to the floor in an untidy heap. Still, at least there was a telly with more than one channel.

We managed to kill a couple of hours in our room before Hayley was wheeled down to theatre. This somewhat scuppered my plans for a crafty lie down once she had gone as they wheeled her down on the bed, leaving me with just the slippery chair. Luckily, I only had to wait a few minutes before I too was called into the little room I had been in before. At least I think it was the same room, but for all I knew they may have had a hundred of these little rooms, each with its own stack of porn and wipe-clean surfaces. This time I admit, I took advantage of the sofa. I sat and tried to relax, thinking positive thoughts about my sperm and all the goodness they had been given over the past two months. I returned to the room shortly before Hayley was wheeled back in. Once we were left alone, she told me that she had had fourteen eggs again. This was excellent news as it meant that every follicle had produced one egg. Admittedly, we did not get to have all of them as we had to give half to our recipient, but it meant that we would all get a good amount to play with. The other good news was that Hayley was nowhere near as uncomfortable as she had been the first time around. Then the bedside phone rang and I heard someone say something to me that I had managed to go thirty-five years without hearing.

'Mr. Saunders? It's the embryologist,' said a voice.

'Yes,' I replied.

'May I just say that you have splendid quality sperm?'

It is not often that I find myself stuck for words but this caught me off guard. The embryologist went on to explain that the count, motility and direction of travel of my sperm were all excellent and far above average. She also confirmed that we would not need ICSI at all and she was happy to pop them in a dish with Hayley's eggs and let them sort things out for themselves. So, fourteen eggs and super sperm! Combine this with the fact that Hayley was now allowed a cup of tea and some toast and you had two very happy people, one of whom was seriously wondering where he could get a 'super-sperm' t-shirt made. The plan was now settled. The sperm and the eggs would be left to make their own introductions, our recipient would be told that she had seven great quality eggs and we got to go home and wait for the call tomorrow regarding how many embryos we had.

We were now in unknown territory, as we had never been in the situation where my sperm were left to fertilise the eggs on their own. Given the officially 'super' nature of them, I had every faith that at least one of them would get its act together, find an egg and do what it should do. That said, it was still a worrying evening. Last time we took it for granted that we would get fertilised embryos as they were being made by a bloke called Steve. This time around there was no such guarantee.

Unlike our first IVF cycle where we got to spend the morning fretting and trying to call the clinic, this time around we got the call exactly when the clinic said we would. It would seem that the embryologists understood that calling when you say you will goes a long way to making people feel at ease with the emotional journey they are going through. Our emotional journey was just about to get a little easier. All seven of Hayley's eggs had fertilised. I shall say that again. All seven. Seven! Brilliant news. It did not mean that all seven would survive though. As I have said before, many people get this far during traditional conception and then have an embryo that fails but they never know about it. We were told that we would get a call the next day and see how many we had that were still looking good.

Once again, the clinic called when they said they would and once again the news was good. All seven were still going strong. This was the point when we had the embryos put back during our first cycle but the clinic we were with now had a policy of waiting until day three to see how the embryos were doing. We would be called the next day in the morning and told what time we had to get down to London to have them put back in, assuming of course, that they all made it through the night once again.

The next day, the clinic called on time again, making it three times in a row. All seven were still going strong so the clinic recommended that we leave them until they reach the blastocyst stage, which should be on day five. We readily agreed and then headed straight for an internet search engine.

When the sperm and the egg first get it together, the resulting embryo doubles its number of cells roughly every day. For the first three days if you look at it under a microscope, it just looks like a circular blob with a bunch of cells in it. Once you get to day four though, things really start happening. Rather than a pile of similar cells, the embryo is now developing two different types of cells. One type is all clustered around the outside of the embryo. These are called the trophoblast. In the centre of the embryo there is now what appears to be a cavity, which is known as a blastocele and is full of the second type of cells. The whole embryo structure is known as a blastocyst. This is a major point in the development of an embryo and once they get to this stage they are far less likely to collapse.

The clinic said that we should leave our embryos in their little culture dish until day five. By this point you can see which bit of the embryo will grow into a baby and which bit will become the placenta. So on the morning of day five we got back into the car and headed for the car park by the hospital. This time there was no posh room with the huge en suite. We were put back into the waiting room and told that we would be called and called we were, exactly when we were told we would be and taken to a little room next to the laboratory. Hayley took a seat in the bed and gave the stirrups a nervous glance while I sat in the traditionally uncomfortable chair. We had a nurse and a doctor in the room with us and once the window on the side wall was opened one of the embryologists poked their head through to say hello and fill us in on what had been going on with our embryos. Of the seven that we had on day three, five had managed to survive until today. This was nothing to worry about as many embryos fail naturally after day three. It did make me think though that when we had the two 'day two' embryos put back on our first cycle, we had assumed that it was Hayley's insides that failed to be sticky enough for both of them to imbed. However, it was more likely that the second embryo simply collapsed by itself a day or so after it was put back. Still, no point in dwelling on that now, we still had five blastocysts that needed our attention. The embryologist said that of the five that were still progressing well, three were looking better than the other two. She suggested that she would pick the best one of the three to put back and look at freezing the other two straight away. The two that were a bit behind, she said, would be monitored for another day and frozen if they caught up.

Blastocyst embryos have a far higher chance of working than day two embryos. As such, UK government recommendations are that only one should be put back at a time. They are only recommendations though and, at the end of the day, it is up to you how many you want to put back. If you have two blastocysts put back then you have about a fifty percent chance of getting pregnant. If you do get pregnant then you have about a fifty percent chance of being pregnant with twins. The government guidelines exist, as twin pregnancies are often more prone to complications and are far more likely to end up with a caesarean section delivery.

As we had the option of picking either one or two of the three best embryos, the staff left us alone for a few minutes to decide what we wanted to do. Obviously we would not be picking which embryos we wanted to put in Hayley but we had to choose if we wanted to go with just the one or go against the government and have the maximum amount of two embryos transferred. It was a tough call to make. If we just had the one put back then there was a fifty percent chance that it would not work and we would always be thinking what if we had put two back and then one may have stuck. However, if we put two back there was a one in three chance that both would stick and we would potentially have twins and all the possible pregnancy complications that could go with it. After a lot of to-ing and fro-ing, we arrived at the decision that the regret of failing with one embryo would outweigh the possible complications of succeeding with two. The doctor returned shortly after we had made our choice and we explained what we wanted to do. He nodded and asked the embryologist to pick the best two for transfer. We had a brief look through the microscope at our two little embryos and the doctor printed us off a picture of them, before they were drawn up into the bendy syringe and inserted back into Hayley's uterus. Once the embryologist had checked the tube to make sure it was empty, the doctor said thank you and goodbye before leaving us to relax for a few minutes before making our way home.

To recap. We now had two embryos somewhere inside Hayley's uterus and three left in their dishes in the laboratory. Of the three that were left, one was doing as well as the two we had just had put back in Hayley, while the other two were a little behind. The embryologist proceeded to cryogenically freeze the one that was doing well and left the other two to their own devises for another twenty-four hours for monitoring. A day later and they had not progressed as we would have hoped and were in fact showing quite major signs of degradation. The embryologist called the next day and explained that the two embryos we had not frozen had turned out not to be viable and that they would be no good to us in the future. As such, they were both left to fade away. The third would stay frozen until such a time that Hayley and I decided what we were going to do with it.

We were now starting the two week wait yet again and that little voice in the back of my head was back. The one that had predicted a success for our first go and a failure for our frozen transfer. This time it was being all positive again, but I decided it was best if I kept the little voice to myself and not complicate matters further. I think that Hayley was feeling quite positive about the impending result too as there were an awful lot of pregnancy tests appearing in the draw. Having had one success, I was of the opinion this treatment was a bonus if it worked: a wonderful bonus admittedly, but still a bonus. As the first week neared its end, my nonchalance was beginning to fade. I was starting to allow myself to think that this really could work which meant if it did not it was going to hurt, although having a toddler running around and attempting to batter your bits does serve as a wonderful distraction from all the waiting.

We made the decision to do the proper test one day before we should have as that day was Mother's Day. We both liked the idea of being able to tell our mothers if it was a positive result on this day of all days. If it was a negative then we could just not mention it. As before, Hayley took the posh digital test into the bathroom and had a wee on it. Also like before it came up positive. We did not know it at the time, but that was where the similarities with Ruby ended.

Two weeks after test day, we went back down to the London clinic to have our official pregnancy scan. They had a very state-of-the-art looking scanner there that could see very tiny embryos and so was perfect for checking what was going on during very early pregnancy.

'And here is baby's heartbeat,' announced the doctor as she manipulated the controls.

Hayley and I both breathed a sigh of relief.

'And here is the other baby's heartbeat,' said the doctor, smiling.

Matilda Beatrice Dawn Saunders
was born on the 24th October 2010 at 08:14
by natural delivery, weighing 4lb 11oz.

George William Robert Saunders
was born on the 24th October 2010 at 08:25
by natural delivery, weighing 5lb 2oz.

Both came home on the 6th November 2010.

9. The negative side of IVF

I have to say that IVF has given Hayley and I something we thought we could never have so I don't really have a bad word to say about it. Sadly though, there are some people who think that IVF and all assisted fertility treatments are bad. If you decide that IVF or something similar is the way for you then you may well encounter one or all of the following arguments against what you are doing.

'It's not natural, is it?'
Well, it rather depends on how you define natural, doesn't it? Natural, as in produced by or existing in nature. Fair enough, that sounds simple enough. IVF does not exist in nature. The tools required couldn't be found growing on a tree no matter how far you go or where you care to look. While we are on the subject though, not much that we use or do in our day-to-day lives fits into that definition. The book you are reading did not occur naturally. The computers that people use, the chairs they sit on, pretty much everything in our lives falls under the broad definition of 'not natural'. Presumably, what people mean by IVF not being natural is that it is not traditional. Traditionally, babies are made between a loving mother and father who make their baby by making love with the lights off and strictly in the missionary position. That would be the traditional way, surely? So what about the babies that are conceived differently? What about the ones that are made when a condom splits between two people who hardly know each other but met under a bus shelter and one thing lead to another? What about the couple who hate each other most of the year but get too drunk over Christmas and end up adding to the already large number of September babies? None of these fit into the bracket of traditional. So whilst IVF is not a traditional method of conception and is as natural as pretty

much everything else in our lives (i.e. not very) it gives couples struggling with fertility a helping hand with conception.

'Infertility is nature's way of controlling the population.'
Well, not really, no. If you look back through nature's history, most of the things that occur to curb the population tend to be localised such as disease outbreaks. If someone says this to you, ask them why Mother Nature, with a whole planet of atoms and molecules to play with, decides the best way of dealing with the ever-increasing population is to give a few people a hard time having babies? Doesn't sound all that likely, does it? To detract slightly more from this argument is the fact that different people go through fertility treatments for different reasons. It may be that you need IVF because you or your partner has a very low sperm count because of a cancer treatment a few years ago. It maybe that your man had the snip when he was with his first wife and now realises that it was not the best thing to have done especially as she ran off with a bloke from Spain who has more sperm that you could ever hope for. Both these, and many more besides, are man-made reasons to have fertility treatment and nothing to do with Mother Nature, bringing doubt to this argument: if the reasons for requiring treatment are made by man, then infertility cannot be nature's way of controlling anything, can it?

'People who have IVF have ugly babies.'
Okay, so I have only ever heard this from one person and she was basing it purely on the fact that she knew people who had IVF and had two unpleasant looking babies. The fact that the couple in question were hardly oil paintings was not important to her argument and she was not going to be swayed with any amount of logic, but I guess it's a case of people fearing that which they do not understand.

'IVF is an affront to God.'

This is a slightly trickier argument to deal with. Applying logic to a theological argument is notoriously difficult. This idea tends to come from only one of the western religions and their argument is based upon the respect for human life that is mentioned a few times in the Bible and other religious texts. The Catholic Bible, for example, claims that life, once conceived, must not be destroyed. Many religious people work on the theory that a fertilised egg is 'alive' whilst some go even further and claim that the egg itself is alive before it even encounters a sperm. Because embryos in IVF that are not viable are left to fade away or are destroyed, the argument from these people is that IVF kills babies. My personal opinion is that nowhere in the Bible does it mention anything about embryo development and when you should class something as being a life, rather than a potential for life. As I said before, logic is not something that can be applied to this argument and it is better to smile sweetly and let people believe whatever they want to believe and to show the kind of respect and tolerance that the Bible teaches towards people with these beliefs.

There are other religious views that IVF is playing God. The theory is that it is God's will that some people cannot have children and it is not for us to challenge this will. Presumably these people felt the same about every little bit of progress that science has made and as such only wear animal skins that they have bred and killed themselves, cut their hair with sharpened rocks and refuse all medical treatment except self-administered and self-grown herbs. They must also believe that someone with cancer should not receive treatment as this is God's will and that pacemakers, hearing aids and even reading glasses are going against what God wants.

On the flip side you can also argue that if God made man, then God is responsible for all that man does, so everything we do and all the progress we make is, in fact, God's will. Best of luck with that one though. That said, there are many religious organisations and believers who have no issues at all with assisted conception and in my opinion these people are to be applauded.

I have to say that although there are groups of people who have beliefs that IVF is a bad thing, pretty much all the individuals that I have met do not voice these opinions. The majority of negative opinions that I have come across has been in the safe and anonymous environment of internet chat rooms, social networking sites or those news programmes that dress up their bigotry as fact and then encourage other equally small minded individuals to make their own knee-jerk reactions on a subject they know little or nothing about. These places are rife with the galloping buffoonery of people who feel that just because a vehicle exists for them to present an opinion, they must be obliged to do so.

I am sure I have come across people who have some or all of these opinions but thankfully none have felt the need to share them with my wife, our children and I.

10. Final thoughts

The main thing to remember about IVF and all assisted conception techniques is that none of the resulting babies happen by accident. No IVF children will ever have to be told by their parents that they were not planned and if Daddy had worn a condom then they would not be here. All IVF children are wanted and planned for, often for many years before they actually arrive. To their parents, they are the most precious things in the whole world.

From my point of view, I look forward to the day that one of our children questions if I am their father. On that day, I can turn to them and say,

'Yes. I have a receipt.'

Top ten tips

1   Research your clinic thoroughly before committing. This can be done by using the information provided by the clinic as well as joining internet groups and forums, talking to people who have had treatment at the clinics you are looking into. You can find good and bad stories about most clinics but at least they are based on first-hand experience.

2   Prepare for each step, i.e. have a list of questions to take to your first appointment.

3   You *can* improve your sperm with vitamins (see page 122).

4   Get quotes for any required drugs. They can often be obtained more cheaply than the clinic supplied ones.

5   Be prepared for your wife/partner to be up and down on an emotional rollercoaster and support her at all times.

6   Remember that you are not alone in either looking into or requiring fertility treatment. A quick stroll around an internet group or two will demonstrate this.

7   Do not worry about things over which you have no control

8   Try to attend as many scans as you can as there are very few times in life when you can look at your lady's insides.

9   Never lose sight of the fact that the end result, assuming everything works, will be a baby. An actual living, breathing, screaming, pooping, puking baby. It is all very well getting excited about the results as you go through treatment but remember the end result and the impact that it could have upon your life.

10 It can be worth it in the end, believe me.

Glossary of medical terms and internet abbreviations

As you trundle through the merry world of infertility, you will come across many and various medical terms and strange abbreviations. If you look for support on one of the numerous internet-based groups or forums, you will find even more. Although this glossary is by no means complete, it should give you enough information to work out what on earth everyone is talking about.

2WW – The two week wait. That time between the embryos going back in and the time when you are officially allowed to take a pregnancy test.

AF / Aunt Flo – A woman's period. Also known as having the painters in, being on the blob or any number of other unpleasant euphemisms.

Baseline scan – Once the female reproductive system has been down regulated, an internal ultrasound scan is performed to check that everything is doing, or not doing, what it should be.

BFN – Big Fat Negative. A negative pregnancy test result.

BFP – Big Fat Positive. A positive pregnancy test result.

Blastocyst – An embryo that is between three and five days old.

DE – Donor Egg. Donated eggs will generally come from someone with a track record of producing good eggs under stimulated conditions. They will be as similar to the recipient as possible.

DH – Darling Husband.

D/R – Down regulation or down regging. The first stage of IVF. Basically the menopause in two weeks.

EC – Egg collection. Removal of matured eggs from the ovaries.

Ectopic pregnancy – It is possible for an egg to fertilise and get stuck in the fallopian tube, which can be very dangerous.

Egg donation – Giving some or all of your eggs to someone who cannot use their own to make babies.

Egg share – Where you donate half your eggs to someone who needs them to conceive.

Embryo – Once an egg is fertilised by a sperm, the resulting cluster of ever multiplying cells is known as an embryo.

ET – Embryo Transfer. Once the sperm and the egg have got together they are popped back into the uterus.

Egg extraction – The process of removing mature eggs from the ovaries.

Fallopian tubes – Connects the ovaries to the uterus. The egg travels down the tubes from the ovary to the uterus.

Fertilisation – When a sperm meets an egg and the two become an embryo.

FET – Frozen embryo transfer. The same as a standard embryo transfer except the embryo has been cryogenically stored beforehand.

Foetus – Six weeks after fertilisation, the embryo has begun developing a spine and nervous system. At this stage it is known as a foetus.

Follicles – Little fluid filled sacks within the ovaries that may contain an egg.

FSH – Follicle stimulating hormone.

GUM clinic – General Urinary Medicine clinic. Formerly known as the clap clinic.

ICSI – Intracytoplasmic sperm injection. Where the sperm is physically injected into the egg to achieve fertilisation.

Medicated cycle – Drugs are used to fool the female body into doing what is required.

Menstrual cycle – Oh for god sake, you know what this is!

Non–medicated cycle – Fertility treatment that is based around the woman's natural cycle.

OHSS – Ovarian Hyper Stimulation Syndrome. Every now and again, the ovaries over-react to the stimulating drugs and start to produce too many follicles. In extreme cases, this may mean stopping the treatment cycle.

OTD – Official test day. The day, two weeks after embryo transfer, when you should do a pregnancy test.

Ovaries – Part of the female reproductive system that contains eggs.

Pessary – A drug taking method that involves inserting the drug in a lower orifice of your choice.

Sperm analysis – The sperm are graded on things like quantity, motility and sense of direction.

Uterus – Also known as the womb. This is where the baby grows if all goes well.

Resources

During our IVF journeys, my wife and I used several websites to obtain information and, more importantly for us, to get in touch with other people going through treatment at the same time as us.

www.fertilityfriends.co.uk
For women and men, mainly UK based. Chat forums on every subject imaginable. This website has been wonderful for us and certainly the one we couldn't have been without during the last 4 years. If you have a question about anything fertility rated then go here first!

www.hfea.gov.uk
The Human Fertilisation & Embryology Authority for the UK. Everything you need to know about treatment options in the UK.

www.advancedfertility.com
Website for the Advanced Fertility Centre of Chicago. Really useful information on all aspects of infertility and IVF treatment, over 200 pages.

www.gettingpregnant.co.uk
Information on causes of infertility, testing and treatment.

www.zitawest.com
According to their website, they are the UK's largest and most successful integrated reproductive health practice, combining the very latest in medical and complementary care.

www.dailystrength.org
A site with support groups on many subjects including infertility. Also has a useful 'ask the experts' section.

www.infertilitynetworkuk.com
Similar to Fertility Friends. Some good articles but it is not free to join.

www.fertilityzone.co.uk
Lots of easy to use forums and discussions. Has an area just for men.

www.fertilityconnect.com
As well as all the usual forums and discussion topics, this also contains some useful articles and links to fertility services.

www.mensfe.net
A website dedicated to male infertility and all it can entail. Features forums, articles, advice and personal stories.

Index